Effective Fraud Control Tactics for Insurers and Managed Care Plans

Daniel R. Anderson
Rick Matarante

Edited By
Nina Youngstrom

Atlantic Information Services, Inc.
1100 17th Street, NW, Suite 300 • Washington, D.C. 20036 • (202) 775-9008

This publication is designed to provide accurate, comprehensive and authoritative information on the subject matter covered. However, the publisher does not warrant that information contained herein is complete or accurate. This book is published with the understanding that the publisher is not engaged in rendering legal or other professional services. If legal advice or other expert assistance is required, the services of a competent professional person should be sought.

ISBN: 0-929156-18-8

Visit the Atlantic Information Services "Health Care Info-Station" at www.aispub.com on the World Wide Web.

For reprint permission, or information regarding individual or bulk purchases, contact: Atlantic Information Services, Inc., 1100 17th Street, NW, Suite 300, Washington, D.C. 20036 (1-800-521-4323; 202-775-9008).

Table of Contents

Preface

For private insurers and managed care plans, implementing a meaningful fraud control strategy is becoming a necessity.

A growing number of states require private carriers to inform the state insurance department of their fraud control plans or, in a few instances, direct insurers to have internal fraud control units, which the private sector calls special investigative units.

Even without regulatory mandates, setting up special investigative units is a sound business strategy. Insurers and managed care plans need to recognize the threat posed by health care fraud, both in terms of civil lawsuits or criminal prosecution, and in terms of getting cheated by their own providers or insureds.

Private fraud control is getting more sophisticated. The authors of this book — the special investigations chief for a managed care company and the former director of a state Medicaid fraud control unit — provide a blueprint for structuring, staffing, and deploying a special investigations unit. The authors also describe how to get management support for the unit, how to train employees in fraud control tactics, and how to network with law enforcement to maximize the unit's impact.

The bottom line: special investigations units are good for *your* bottom line. If your unit is effective, its value will be proven many times over, by the money insurers and managed care plans save in detecting fraud schemes before they inflict too much damage, by deterring providers from bad acts when they see a colleague go down, and by recovering money in civil lawsuits or criminal prosecutions.

About the Authors

Daniel R. Anderson is formerly an assistant attorney general for the state of Maryland and director of that state's Medicaid fraud control unit, where he prosecuted numerous health care providers for fraud and abuse. Anderson has a law degree from the University of Baltimore. Last year, he was awarded the John B. Pickett Fellowship at Harvard University's John F. Kennedy School of Government, where he earned a master's degree in public administration, specializing in health care policy.

Rick Matarante is manager of the special investigations unit at Oxford Health Plans, Inc., where he and his four staff members opened more than 600 cases in their first year of operation. He was formerly the manager of the provider/employee investigation team at Blue Cross Blue Shield of New Jersey.

CHAPTER 1

Overview: Fighting Health Fraud

Never before has it been more critical for health care providers and insurers to contain costs. In the private sector, an increasingly competitive marketplace and the advent of capitated payments have forced the price of many health care services down to a level at which costs are barely recouped. In the public sector, political concerns militate against increased expenditures for Medicare, Medicaid, and other government-sponsored health plans, yet sustaining the same level of medical services practically demands more spending.

One method of reducing health care costs which has proven effective is more aggressive prevention and detection of wasteful, fraudulent, and abusive activities. In a health care system where the availability of services directly correlates to a finite resource base, every dollar lost to such malfeasance affects the ability of providers and insurers to provide and pay for additional services. As proof of this, look at the experience of several states which now have either cut, or have considered reducing, available services to their Medicaid recipients due to dwindling funds and skyrocketing costs. Therefore, effective fraud prevention and detection is now a high priority for both insurers and providers.

The health care industry in this country has become a booming business. It is estimated that in 1996, Americans will spend over $1 trillion dollars to obtain health care from varied sources within the United States. This number represents nearly 16% of our gross national product and, despite some recent trends indicating a slight decline in expenditures, concerns about cost are paramount.

The federal and state governments pay nearly 35% of the nation's health care bill, and costs are rising fastest for them. The Medicaid program, for example, which was established in 1965 to provide health care to the indigent, has seen enrollment explode.

State expenditures for Medicaid have doubled in the past five years, and in some urban areas, such as Baltimore and New York, it is not uncommon for one-fourth of the population to rely on Medicaid for basic health needs. Even though Medicaid is funded 50% by federal money, several states now spend between 15% and 20% of their general budget to sustain the program.

As our population ages, enrollment in the Medicare program has similarly increased, costing the federal government billions of dollars each year. The trust fund from which a large portion of Medicare expenditures come is expected to be depleted in the first decade of the new millennium. Containing health care costs is not solely a government concern. Indeed, given the increasing competitive forces within the private health care sector, controlling costs has become a primary concern of both insurers and health care providers.

It is against this backdrop that fraudulent and abusive activities within the health care sector have garnered greater attention. According to sources as varied as the General Accounting Office and the U.S. Chamber of Commerce, fraud and abuse by health care providers and related service providers eat up between 10% and 15% of all health care expenditures. A report issued in 1994 by the then-minority staff of the United States Senate Special Committee on Aging estimated that for the past five years, losses from health care fraud and abuse totaled about $418 billion, or about four times as much as the entire savings and loan crisis has cost this country to date. Even assuming a more optimistic estimate, these losses not only threaten the continued ability of government to provide comparable levels of service in the future, they also dampen the ability of health care providers to compete in today's marketplace.

The Justice Department has made health care fraud enforcement a top priority, just behind violent crime. The Federal Bureau of Investigation has similarly beefed up its efforts in this area and has increased its caseload dramatically. In 1991, the FBI had only 365 pending health care fraud investigations, yet by the end of 1993 that number had nearly tripled to 1,051 pending investigations. Additional FBI agents are being assigned each year to investigate this kind of crime.

The Office of Inspector General of the Department of Health and Human Services has nearly 400 staff nationwide assigned to detecting fraud against Medicare, Medicaid and certain other government insurance programs. The Health Care Financing Administration has established Medicare fraud and abuse units in its carriers and intermediaries across the country, and has recently gone online with the Fraud Investigations Database. Investigative agents of the Inspector General of Amtrak, CHAMPUS, and the United States Postal Inspection Service have all joined the fight against health care fraud within their respective programs.

New Law Empowers Fraud Enforcement

A new health insurance reform law, the Health Insurance Portability and Accountability Act of 1996, has allocated even more funding for the government's war on fraud, and the Inspector General has already vowed to use some of the funds to set up more offices and agents to fight fraud. Also, the new law assures a steady supply of funds from the new fraud and abuse control account, which lets the government recycle fines and penalties from successful fraud prosecutions to make additional cases (see Chapter 11).

The new insurance reform law also serves up a number of powerful fraud fighting tools. Among them: a new crime of health fraud; a new "intermediate sanction" for transgressing Medicare HMOs; and higher civil money penalties, which the government can levy for health fraud.

On the state level, virtually every state now has a Medicaid fraud control unit charged with detecting and prosecuting health care providers who cheat the Medicaid program. Mainly, these units are incorporated into state attorneys general offices, though in some instances are placed within the jurisdiction of the state police, state auditor or other state agencies. Collectively, the units have obtained over 7,000 convictions of corrupt health care providers and vendors, such as laboratories and transportation companies.

The private sector is increasingly taking note of health care fraud and abuse occurring within that sector. The National Health Care Anti-Fraud Association includes members from the insurance industry, private health care providers, and law enforcement agencies concerned with this crime. The collective experiences of both the law enforcement community and the private sector has provided both the impetus and the knowledge necessary for private concerns to establish their own internal investigations unit.

In light of these factors, there's great urgency for providers and insurers to establish internal fraud and abuse control units, usually referred to as "special investigations units (SIUs)" in the private sector.

Not only do internal investigation units assist in determining what potential fraud has been committed against the insurer, internal investigation units established by insurers and managed care plans can perform several other functions. For example, a well-designed internal investigation unit can help health plans avoid prosecutions in civil, criminal or administrative proceedings; can mitigate damages and penalties and institute corrective actions; can reduce the liability of officers, directors and employees; and can support corporate actions in disciplining or discharging employees, medical staff members, or directors.

There are two approaches to fraud control: reactive and proactive. Reactive fraud control, also known as "pay and chase," occurs after the claims are submitted for payment by a health care provider and, often, have been paid. Sometimes phony claims are relatively easy to spot, such as those filed on behalf of men alleged to have received a hysterectomy, infants receiving vision tests, drug addicts alleged to be getting both methadone and abusable drugs, members of the same family all receiving prescriptions for the same abusable drugs, utilization by patients receiving abusable drugs from disparate pharmacies throughout various parts of a city, and laboratory tests which are "unbundled" in order to maximize reimbursement. All these nonsensical claims merit greater review by health care professionals and utilization review specialists.

There is a tendency in the private sector to leave this task of claims review to individuals whose sole training and responsibility is to input data contained on billing invoices. All too often, the primary concern of payers is that health care providers get paid quickly and that information entered into the insurers' database is an accurate reflection of the information contained on the billing invoice. Likewise, incentives are provided to employees to process claims both quickly and accurately, with accuracy defined as a correct reflection of the information contained on the claims submission and not of the underlying service on which the claim is based. There is not much motivation for employees to question the underlying basis for the submitted invoice. That would slow down claims processing, arousing the ire of the provider awaiting payment and the claims processing department supervisor seeking to achieve an established goal of the number of claims to be processed within a given month.

Claims review is one area where the government deserves credit for leading the way. The Medicaid program, for example, has always aggressively deployed its Surveillance and Utilization Review Subsystem to detect suspicious claims. This system remains state-of-the-art in many states in comparing providers to their professional peers to catch aberrant billing patterns. Providers within the same specialty and geographic area are compared to each other and when one bills excessively, the computer notes it. This does not mean that an aberrant health care provider is immediately referred for criminal investigation. Indeed, a very low percentage of health care providers detected by this computer system are referred for criminal prosecution.

Nevertheless, once an anomalous billing pattern is established, trained medical professionals employed by the Medicaid program will either review the claim submissions or will request further information from the provider to determine the underlying basis for the claims. For example, a Boston dentist will be compared to other dentists treating the Medicaid population in Boston. When the particular dentist's billing patterns suddenly appear excessive compared to his or her fellow dentists within that geographic area, the Surveillance and Utilization Review Subsystem will so indicate. Medicaid personnel will then review the various facts presented by the claims submissions of the suspect dentist. This review will determine whether there is a rational explanation for aberrant billing patterns or whether fraudulent activities warrant further investigation. For example, the state may find that a dentist who bills an excessive number of amalgams is located next to a children's clinic, which would explain why more amalgams are billed by the dentist compared to peers who treat older populations.

Of course, systems such as the Surveillance and Utilization Review Subsystem require advanced information technology. Patterns of fraud must first be formulated by experienced investigators working in tandem with health care professionals, and an information system must be structured which recognizes those patterns. Again, the Medicaid program has substantial experience in this area and can provide useful information to insurers and managed care plans considering a similar program.

Unfortunately, these obvious, easier-to-detect kinds of frauds — what professionals in the field call self-revealing frauds — are less common than the confounding, hard-to-detect kinds of frauds. That's why it is absolutely vital that an investigator have a working knowledge of the nature of the health care industry and those areas which are most vulnerable to fraud and abuse.

One great way to keep abreast of developments in fraud and abuse is getting the "fraud alerts" issued by the office of inspector general, Department of Health and Human Services. These alerts contain the latest information obtained by the office of inspector general concerning health care fraud schemes uncovered across the nation.

Private Payers Should Stress Prevention

Obviously, from the perspective of one who is paying the bill, fraud *prevention* should take precedence over fraud *detection*. Toward that end, Medicare recently started verifying that health care providers actually had a physical address before sending checks and payments to those providers — something insurers should also do. As simple as this may sound, rarely have insurers undertaken an independent investigation to determine whether a health care provider actually existed.

This lack of basic verification leads to a number of cases in which individuals attempting to cheat Medicare (and, undoubtedly, other insurers) merely established post office box addresses and submitted fraudulent claims. Assuming claims submitted by these scam artists made it through the claims process, reimbursement checks would then be mailed to the post office box, the fraudulent providers would get the money and disappear — leaving little hope for recovery. Now, Medicare verifies that the provider actually has an office and is rendering medical services at the location indicated.

An important adjunct to this verification is making sure that appropriate personnel are employed by the health care provider to actually render the level of care for which it is billing. The Medicaid program has recently witnessed so-called hit and run schemes in which non-health care professionals run advertisements in local newspapers, claiming to be physicians setting up local clinics. These ads solicited the resumes of physicians to be employed by the clinic and, during bogus hiring interviews, the potential physician/employees were asked to provide information, such as their Medicaid or Medicare provider identification numbers. This information, together with the data on a typical resume, allowed the con artist to submit claims bearing that physician's number under the aegis of the sham clinic. By the time such a fraud is detected, zealous cheats were able to steal hundreds of thousands of dollars with little hope of recovery. It is therefore vital that insurers verify that the health care provider submitting bills is the one actually rendering the services.

Insurers also need to verify that the provider has sufficient expertise and equipment to provide the level of care for which bills are submitted. A health care provider billing for sophisticated blood tests or other services for which he or she is either not trained or not appropriately equipped should immediately raise red flags. Once again, cooperation with the appropriate licensing authorities should assist in making such determinations. In addition, most legitimate health care providers are more than willing to allow access to their offices to make a quick review of the equipment and supplies they have on hand. Generally, only those providers with something to conceal would hesitate to provide such limited and unobtrusive access.

A good fraud investigator makes it his or her business to routinely scan local and community newspapers to see whether health care providers are advertising for "special" services. While health care providers are certainly guaranteed the freedoms granted to most of us to advertise in these journals and generally are free to do so in an unregulated fashion, there are certain indicators that should interest a fraud investigator. For example, any health care provider offering something of value to patients in return for their patronage is suspect. One New York podiatrist was prosecuted by state authorities after it was learned he offered free tennis shoes to his patients in return for their patronage. Another pled guilty after luring patients with free chinese food.

Why are such rebates suspect? From a purely economic standpoint, health care providers who offer such incentives may recoup the cost of those incentives by padding bills submitted to the insurers. The podiatrist offering free tennis shoes to his patients, for example, had every incentive to bill for additional services over and above those medically necessary for the patient — which he did. Such an incentive also causes patients to seek care which they may not need. Patients in New York, for example, may not have needed podiatry care, but they wanted new tennis shoes and therefore sought out the podiatrist willing to provide them — at taxpayer expense!

Another indication of possible fraud in such advertisements occurs when health care providers advertise that they specialize in "accident" cases or personal injury claims. Again, that is not to say that all doctors who provide this service are committing fraud. Nonetheless, an insurer would be well-advised to carefully scrutinize claims originating from such an office, particularly bearing in mind that legal settlements in such cases are calculated based upon a multiple of the health claims submitted. This causes great pressure from a variety of sources for the provider to increase both the number and the level of claimed services, often at the expense of the insurer.

Patients often constitute the first line of defense against fraud. An activist health care consumer will question both the cost and the medical necessity of provided services, causing an otherwise profligate provider to more reasonably bill his or her services. That's why it's helpful to send all patients explanation of medical benefits letters, when economically feasible, to make it as simple as possible for patients to report allegations of fraud and abuse. Many insurers have established a fraud hotline, usually offering patients a toll-free, 800 number they can call to anonymously report allegations of malfeasance.

One important caveat to the use of explanation of benefits forms: Responding to complaints which arise only through beneficiaries can sometimes cause the insurer's internal investigation unit to be solely reactive, dissuading investigations into larger patterns of fraud and abuse. Rather than focusing on fraud control, the internal investigations unit may instead focus instead on disposing of cases.

In a related matter, it is vital that at the point at which the insurer determines that a possible fraud occurred, patients must be contacted to determine what (if any) services were in fact rendered by the suspect provider. While patients are not always the best historians of their own care, their eventual input in an investigation is vital. In the event of a trial against the provider, jurors always want to know what care the patients received and whether the patients were pleased with that care.

Coordination among various insurers (including Medicare and Medicaid) is an invaluable resource in conducting an investigation. It has been the experience of fraud investigators that a health care provider who is stealing from one insurer is almost certainly stealing from others. If Medicaid has been the victim of a crime, it is likely that same provider is also stealing from private insurers.

Several resources in this area are particularly valuable. The National Health Care Anti-Fraud Association in Washington, D.C., is devoted to coordinating anti-fraud activities among private and government payers. Using the association's services, you can contact insurers nationwide and receive timely information indicating whether a provider you suspect of wrongdoing has committed similar acts against other insurers.

In addition, you can contact your state Medicaid fraud control unit for coordinating efforts involving possible fraud against the

Medicaid program. These units are now located in 48 states, typically in the office of the state attorney general. By revealing the evidence of your investigation, you may determine that the Medicaid program has been similarly victimized by a crime. If that is the case, the Medicaid fraud control unit may be willing to seek authority from the Department of Health and Human Services to append your claims involving private insurance fraud to those involving any fraud against the Medicaid program in a criminal or civil action it can maintain in state court.

The main Justice Department and many United States attorneys' offices throughout the country have attorneys and prosecutors devoted solely to investigating health care fraud allegations. Coordinating with the local office of the FBI or directly contacting the U.S. Attorney in your state may prove beneficial in case the insurance fraud exceeds a minimal amount set by your local jurisdiction for litigation.

Maintaining liaison with other insurers or managed care plans is extremely helpful. Your unit does not want to inadvertantly disrupt an ongoing investigation by settling an issue that your state's Medicaid fraud control unit has under investigation. By working with the state, private insurers also can learn about the schemes used by the provider community (and often broadcast through their networking efforts). And, for example, if you are investigating a psychiatric provider who has billed you for 12 hour-long visits in one day, it would be important to learn that she has also billed another insurer for additional hours on the same day, or is about to have her license suspended by the state.

Access to the Internet and national health care prosecution databases is also a plus. The insurer's SIU computers should be equipped with modems and software. On-line access to insurers' paid claims data is the standard, but a software program that permits the agent to meld parallel queries — for example, locate any beneficiaries seen by all of a group of providers suspected of ping-ponging patients — is even better. Although the software is within the budgetary reach of most SIUs, the cost of on-line time for using such programs can be prohibitive, and improperly trained personnel have been known to initiate requests that crash the system.

Notwithstanding the need for information and the benefits of networking, your investigative unit should be aware of and careful about confidentiality regarding patient information. Greater public uproar about the casual "sale" of patient information is making insurers into the bad guys when it comes to patient privacy.

Make sure that your inquiries are fully legal and that you are aware of and honor all legal and ethical privileges. Federal laws and regulations are particularly strict when it comes to using information in mental health records or on drug and alcohol rehabilitation services (42 CFR 290dd and 42 CFR 290ee).

CHAPTER 2

Reasons to Start a Special Investigations Unit

The most compelling reason to start a special investigations unit (SIU) is financial. Through its investigation and enforcement efforts, SIUs can serve as a tourniquet on the fraud and abuse-induced hemorrhaging of money from insurers. SIUs accomplish this through prevention and deterrence — by stopping providers and others from manipulating money out of the system — and through recovery of lost funds. Most companies are going to judge their SIUs by comparing the savings to the cost of the unit.

With 10% of health care expenditures wasted on fraud and abuse, calculate what that would mean to your company over a year's time and you will understand the magnitude of the possible loss — and see a persuasive reason to start up or strengthen an SIU. Insurers and health plans also have a responsibility to their premium payers. Employers and individuals are paying more and more money to receive insurance and in many instances getting less and less. It's very important to show your customers that your company is making a good-faith effort to protect those premium dollars and to ensure they are used to underwrite medical care — not to line the pockets of the unscrupulous. Insureds also favorably perceive a health plan that does its part to control the rising cost of health care.

Insurers and health plans have a responsibility to protect premium payers beyond finances. With the push towards managed care, insurers have an obligation to ensure that their network of providers are of the highest quality — and aren't cheats. There have been a few instances where providers who are committing fraud put their greed ahead of the patient's welfare.

Another reason to start SIUs is the business-world's version of keeping up with the Joneses. Even a decade ago, not many companies had SIUs, or they were very small. Now, SIUs are getting more prevalent — even being advertised on radio and television.

SIUs also are a boon for marketing purposes. In some circumstances, an SIU may be the feature that gets a health plan a contract within an industry with very competitive pricing. Benefits coordinators may choose your company over another because they know about your cost-containment measures. Also, an SIU can be a source of favorable publicity, which is always an effective marketing tool.

Soon, an insurer and managed care plan may have no choice but to start an SIU as regulators get more active in private-insurance fraud control. Twenty-nine states have established insurance fraud bureaus, and that number will continue to grow. Ten states require insurance carriers to have plans to detect and prevent fraud, and five states actually mandate SIUs. Consult the regulations for your type of business to determine if you are in a state requiring special fraud control efforts.

CHAPTER **3**

Setting Up a Special Investigations Unit

When you set out to organize your special investigations unit (SIU), many questions will arise: Where and who should the SIU report to? How many people do I hire? Whom do I hire? How will I generate cases? Do I need a hotline?

To start, an SIU must have a philosophy. What kind of fraud unit will it be? Will it emphasize the pursuit of financial recoveries, or mainly refer cases for government prosecutions? Will the SIU be made up predominantly of desk investigators or on-the-street investigators? Will it work with outside agencies, or keep cases internal? These philosophies should be discussed with your corporate legal department before initiating the SIU.

Another key decision is the location of the SIU in the insurer or managed care plan. There is no ideal place to locate the SIU. Regardless of where it winds up, it's critical to establish and maintain good relationships with other areas.

Among the choices of locations for the SIU:

- Audit department: The benefits of being tied into the audit department are that similarity of functions and the additional resources to tap when needed, especially for internal cases.
- Legal department: The benefits here stem from the obvious legal ramifications of health fraud cases. If the legal area has litigators, latch onto them.
- Claims processing: Locating the SIU within the claims department has appeal because most of its work revolves around the actual claims.

The placement of the SIU may also depend upon whether the unit is responsible for policing fraud perpetrated by the insurer. Providers often develop relationships with persons in the claims department — some good, some bad. If the job of the SIU is to identify kickbacks, employee misconduct, or other inappropriate arrangements within the insurer, then the SIU should be isolated, both spatially and as to chain of command, from the operational functions of the insurer.

The SIU as in-house intelligence is perhaps more important in the managed care setting. Many of the risk-sharing structures found in managed care systems are conducive to in-house problems. The fact that a managed care patient has less choice in the care provided and the person providing it means that someone within the managed care organization has more. This can be problematic.

For example, a primary care physician who is paid on a capitated basis might not hesitate to befriend an employee who is responsible for referring patients in the hope of getting the healthier patients in exchange for simple friendship, baseball tickets or cash.

In such cases, isolation of the SIU is an advantage in conducting a meaningful inquiry into the insurer's own activities. The disadvantages of segregation, however, include mistrust of the unit by operational employees; jealousy of perceived privileges; and a resulting lack of cooperation and referrals from in-house sources.

Selecting your staff is probably the most important part of starting up a new fraud control unit. Who to hire — and how many — are critical questions to answer correctly. There generally are going to be many cases referred to the SIU initially. With a small starting staff, you need to make sure you don't fall too far behind at the onset. Try to find hardworking, self-motivated, and efficient people to try and stay on top of the cases.

Here are key positions to fill when forming an SIU:

Fraud analysts. Regardless of how many people you hire to start up, one of them must be an analyst. In most SIUs, fraud analyst is the most important position. Analysts provide investigators with a preliminary analysis of a case so the investigator can jump right into the investigation portion of the case. This will allow the investigator to be able to conduct multiple investigations at the same time. Also, analysts open the door for people within your organization to work with the SIU when that might not have otherwise been possible. This will allow you the opportunity to hire people with good claims backgrounds, but not necessarily investigation backgrounds.

The functions of fraud analysts are numerous. They include:

(1) Collecting, collating, analyzing and interpreting data, both internally and externally;

(2) Assisting the investigators in gathering the documentation needed to conduct an investigation;

(3) Controlling and maintaining departmental data in an organized manner; and

(4) Preserving confidentiality.

Investigators/senior investigators. While these positions are similar, an SIU may make a distinction based on experience, salary ranges, and opportunity for upward mobility. Basically, investigators will be performing the same jobs, but you might want to set aside the more complex or sensitive cases for the senior investigators.

The functions of investigators may include:

(1) Detecting fraudulent activity;

(2) Organizing the investigations;

(3) Securing information;

(4) Preparing reports of investigations; and

(5) Conducting settlement negotiations.

Your investigative staff will work with law enforcement personnel, when applicable. Their job will be to prove or disprove the existence of fraud.

Supervisors. Depending on the structure of the company and the way your own time is divided, you could have an assistant manager, manager and/or director, or any combination of the three. This person would be responsible for:

(1) Coordinating similar investigations;

(2) Assigning the cases to the investigators;

(3) Monitoring the progress of the investigations;

(4) Setting the direction for the unit;

(5) Training the SIU personnel; and

(6) When possible, helping with the investigations.

In house attorneys. Although many SIUs operate successfully without the benefit of an in-house attorney, the SIU should consider hiring an attorney with prosecutorial experience, preferably in fraud. In addition to being helpful with privilege and evidentiary issues, the attorney can often define a worthwhile criminal case at an early stage of the investigation, thus saving the SIU time and effort. In addition, an experienced litigator will have credibility with government prosecutors and may be able to assist in establishing liaisons necessary to the acceptance of referrals to government authorities.

Significantly, the "strike force" concept of joining attorneys with auditors and investigators has been used in Medicaid fraud control units for more than fifteen years.

An attorney should also be integrally involved in establishing the chain of custody for evidence to be used in prosecution efforts, including controls for using electronic data. Chain of custody issues become extraordinarily complicated when a provider's electronic data is manipulated for use in preparing trial exhibits. The SIU does not want to find itself in front of a jury without any admissible evidence on the provider's fraudulent billings.

Clerical workers and computer programmers. SIUs also need the assistance of clerical staff and computer programmers. With the number of reports that will be needed, programmers will help with ordering and compiling the data. And in terms of clerical workers, SIUs need people to input the case data onto a database, be in charge of the hotline and serve as office manager. Notwithstanding the importance of these two job categories, they are not necessary for a start-up operation for those facing very tight budgets.

Types of Cases Affect Skills Needed

When hiring, try to determine what kinds of cases you will predominantly get. For example, if your cases will mostly be procedure-type cases, recruit someone comfortable working with medical procedures and terminologies.

If your cases involve eligibility issues, consider someone with underwriting experience or someone with an understanding of underwriting regulations and/or contractual language. However, if the types of cases your SIU will face are unclear, take advantage of the great resources right in your company. Because most of the work will involve claims, hire someone who has a lot of claims experience and understands the payment system and the different benefits, though these candidates will most likely lack investigative skills.

Some experts prefer to hire an internal person for the analyst position. Promoting an investigator to analyst may be wise. If you are inclined to hire outside of your organization, look for law enforcement, investigative or insurance backgrounds. People with experience tend to cost a little more, so it is important to keep in line with your budget and maximize your resources. Consider hiring people with limited experience, and then playing the role of the experienced investigator. It's often easier to teach someone how to be an investigator than it is to teach someone about insurance. If the money is available, get at least one experienced person into the group, which will let the director perform his or her own administrative duties.

It is very important that insurers train their investigators well and that these investigators be trained to ask the correct questions when interviewing providers. In any investigation involving health care fraud, some of the most pertinent information to be derived will come directly from the mouth of the health care provider under investigation. This requires investigators to possess a modicum of medical knowledge, the ability to be assertive in a difficult situation, and the ability to be flexible when the situation may change. For example, it is not uncommon for health care providers to want to provide an explanation for unmasked aberrant-billing patterns.

Investigators should be trained to listen very carefully to what is said, make careful notes of the conversation, and ask the appropriate questions for the circumstances.

A well trained investigator will allow the provider to speak freely and without challenge or interruption to derive as much information as possible without being too confrontational. Obviously, a confrontational approach could result in the health care provider refusing to speak further and seeking legal counsel, at which point all direct contact with the provider will likely cease.

During the course of such a discussion, the investigator should be trained to ask such non-threatening and seemingly innocuous questions as the number of employees employed by the physician and the extent to which the physician employs them. For example, an office that bills for a high volume of patients may have only one physician's assistant or other physician extender. If the investigator can get the physician to state employment information on the record, such an admission may later prove valuable in a trial challenging the number of services billed. An investigator should also be able to determine quite easily the type of machinery, equipment and supplies utilized by the provider.

When looking within the company for an investigator, try to find someone with:

- Experience in the medical profession;
- Utilization review or medical management sophistication;
- Claims experience (auditory preferred); and
- Good investigative skills.

Among external candidates, seek experience within the medical or an investigative profession or hire someone with a law enforcement background.

To Investigate Claimants, Know Claims Payment Systems, Benefits

The intricacies of staffing takes a more complex turn depending on the kinds of fraud investigations the SIU undertakes. For example, when conducting provider investigations, the investigative qualities of your agents should include:

- Knowledge/experience with medical terminology.
- Knowledge/experience with CPT-4 and ICD-9 codes.
- Experience in communicating with providers.
- Knowledge of claims payment system and company benefits.

When undertaking investigations of claimants, investigative qualities should include knowledge of claims payment systems and benefits and with good investigative skills, including perhaps a claims investigator. If you go outside for this person, look for a law enforcement background or other experience in the investigative profession.

When taking on eligibility investigations, investigative qualities should include knowledge of underwriting regulations; experience with contracts; and good negotiating skills. If you plan to hire from within, look for someone from the underwriting area or contract development area.

Finally, when the SIU takes on suspected fraud within its own insurance company or managed care plan, it's vital to use an investigator with extensive investigative experience, tremendous discretion, an understanding of basic audit procedures, and knowledge of corporate policies and procedures. Such investigators should be among your existing employees, but if you have to go outside, seek someone with strong investigative skills.

CHAPTER 4

Building a Caseload

Building the caseload is another big challenge for the special investigations unit (SIU). There are different ways of building a caseload and assorted tools to be used under varying circumstances. Part of this process is conducting awareness training for the company to ensure cases are referred to the SIU. The SIU's job is to identify as much fraud as possible and the best way to do that is to encourage as many referrals as possible.

At first cases will start to trickle in. This will serve as a crystal ball for the types of cases you are going to see and also indicate what the company believes is fraud.

Consider putting together a program of fraud awareness training for the entire company. Every employee should be made aware of the problem of fraud and how it relates to them. Employees are also customers of the insurance or managed care plan. If you have to prioritize training, it is more important to meet initially with the operations area, which deals mostly with claims. Most referrals to the SIU will come from operations.

The goals of these training sessions are to introduce your unit to the company; explain what fraud is; relay any regulatory requirements (i.e. mandatory referrals of fraud cases to state insurance fraud bureaus); and get employees pumped up to refer cases to you. This can be accomplished by offering up examples of cases that have been investigated in the past.

Training should have three stages:

- ***Phase 1: An introductory session.*** Many employees won't realize the company has an SIU. Define fraud, and explain the reasons for the SIU — providing examples of health care fraud cases, perhaps even telling horror stories. Let them know that the success of any SIU depends on them. They are the eyes and ears of the fraud unit.

- *Phase 2:* Once current employees have been trained, provide a condensed version for new employees at orientation. This will ensure the entire company gets fraud awareness training.
- *Phase 3:* Once the SIU establishes some cases, periodically update the awareness training. During this phase, provide examples of the types of fraud the SIU is uncovering and thank those who have referred cases to you.

Historically, departments that have received fraud awareness training will begin to refer cases. These employees tend to look at the claims a little closer than before and will find possible problems they wouldn't have flagged before. Re-educate departments when referrals stop flowing from them.

In addition to employee referrals, another effective method to build the SIU's caseload is through developing or purchasing outside computer software designed to detect fraudulent activity. These types of programs use your paid-claims history to establish patterns and trends, giving indicators of possibly fraudulent perpetrators. The SIU will glean targets to investigate without the need of a referral from outside sources. That will give you the capability of being proactive while increasing your caseload.

Being proactive has become a very important challenge for SIUs. Executives realize fraud is out there and they want it stopped on a pre-payment basis. Having software define patterns can allow for investigations to be completed before the financial loss has been too great.

Today, there are many companies marketing fraud detection software. SIUs should compare them to the capabilities of your in-house systems. Considerations should include cost; compatibility; turn-around time for data; and confidence in data.

Establishing a Database

Another big caseload-building challenge for an SIU is establishing a database. Having a database can serve multiple purposes. First, it is a way to keep track of cases and maintain cases in an organized manner. Secondly, SIU supervisors will be able to keep a handle on all of the cases and assign the new cases in an equitable manner. Third, it will help SIU directors meet demands for statistics on the progress of the unit. The database will make it easier to prepare statistics in a timely and accurate manner, and in whatever format you choose.

Once enough data is input into the database, SIU staff can use this information to identify problem areas. For example, you may identify problems within a specialty in a certain location that needs a closer look, or you may identify multiple cases with the same or similar addresses, which may change the complexion of the case. Whatever the circumstances are, a database is another way of beefing up the SIU caseload.

Finally, the use of a hotline or post office box will almost assuredly increase the volume of work. SIUs trying to build a caseload without getting overwhelmed, but lacking the manpower to staff a hotline, should perhaps consider having a separate post office box or Internet address for subscribers or providers to use to refer alleged cases of fraud to the department. The SIU would send an informational certificate inside explanation of benefits forms. This certificate would give generic examples of fraudulent activity and instruct potential referrers to document the details of their case in writing and mail it to the post office box or transmit it.

The disadvantage of such an approach is the loss of legitimate referrals because a patient lacks the desire to take time to put everything in writing or is uncomfortable putting a complaint in writing. On the other hand, because writing is a deterrent to referrals, the SIU will have a built-in control on the amount of referrals, which will keep a fledgling SIU from becoming overwhelmed.

A post office box is also a screening device. Anyone who takes the time to put a complaint in writing is more likely to have a valid complaint. Plus, using a post office box means it's unlikely the SIU will have to waste its energy sorting through routine, misdirected customer service complaints.

The alternative is setting up an anonymous hotline to take reports of suspicions of fraud. There are a couple of strategies that can be employed when using a hotline:

- The most common hotline set-up involves having the calls come directly into the SIU and having them answered by either departmental operators or investigative staff. That gives the SIU control over the calls, which enables you to secure any additional information you may need right then and to transfer non-fraud related issues to the proper department. Unfortunately, hot lines demand a lot of staff time — to treat the caller properly and handle follow-up calls — which is something the SIU may not have.
- Have hotline calls go into the customer service line by creating a touch-tone prompt specifically for fraud. That eliminates SIU staff-drain because the customer service function is already in place. Also, there should be few customer service related issues

because the prompt will direct the calls to the appropriate line. But the SIU gives up control of the case and has to educate the customer service people.

- Have calls go directly into the unit on a separate phone line. All calls will be answered by an automated answering system. That gives the SIU control over cases, responding to the referral at a pace that fits into its schedule and screening the calls to accept only fraud related referrals. Disadvantages, however, would include a possible increase in customer service calls and the risk of not being able to identify an anonymous caller.

Which choice your SIU makes depends on budgetary and workload considerations. Some experts lean toward the automated answering system because the SIU gets plenty of referrals and can take all of them, but can respond as time and workload allows.

An increased caseload validates the need for an SIU. The more cases you can look through, the better the chances of finding those big dollar cases — and perpetuating upper management support.

CHAPTER 5

Education and Deterrence

Special investigations units (SIU) in the health care industry is one of the few enforcement units that will frequently pull its weight financially. An established SIU will generally recover enough money every year to pay for the cost of the unit's operation. The emphasis which many companies place on the financial savings, however, often eclipses other important functions of the unit — education and deterrence. They accomplish the less-easily measured goal of preventing fraud and abuse before they become a drain on the company's resources. Although it may be more difficult to measure the success of education and deterrence, they are important and need to be considered when setting forth the criteria and standards which the SIU is expected to meet.

In these days of severe budget constraints and corporate downsizing, the fraud detection staffs of private insurers are often the first affected by budget cutbacks. They frequently are considered the stepchildren to the seemingly more important task of timely and accurate claims processing. Private insurers are increasingly recognizing, however, that the activities of fraud detection within their organizations has a ripple effect by not only recovering money actually stolen, but also deterring other providers from engaging in similar activities. This has also been the experience of law enforcement professionals assigned to combating Medicare and Medicaid fraud.

Although hundreds of millions of dollars are recovered each year by these authorities as a result of their successful fraud investigations, the fruits of these investigations are much higher because each publicized case deters countless other providers from engaging in fraudulent activities. While this number is difficult to quantify, law enforcement authorities can attest to this effect through actual experience.

For example, during the course of one state Medicaid fraud control unit's undercover investigation, investigators posing as patients were physically present in a physician's office when they heard him discussing an article from that day's newspaper on the conviction of a provider committing a similar type of fraud for which this MD was under investigation. The provider being probed immediately ceased his fraudulent billing based solely on publicity about a similar investigation.

Repeated studies have shown that white collar criminals are particularly susceptible to general deterrence. It is well-established that professionals in the health care field remain very aware of such occurrences within their profession. Actions taken by either law enforcement or by insurance companies against providers are usually well-publicized within the profession and have an immeasurable effect upon health care providers.

Lack of Education Spurs Fraud

Education is a powerful tool in fraud deterrence and prevention. One of the most expensive lessons of inadequate education about health care fraud involves the laboratory industry's decision to market expensive, exotic tests with basic panels. In one highly publicized case, a testing lab deceived doctors into thinking that the added exotics were essentially free, when in fact the added tests were billed to insurers at $10 or $20 or more. Physicians checked off a box on the laboratory requisition form each time they needed a basic panel, often not noticing that the panel contained unnecessary, "free" extras. Laboratories defended the billings for the medically unnecessary exotics by pointing to the fact that the physician had ordered the profile, even though the physicians were essentially tricked into ordering the exotic tests.

Over the years and throughout the industry, this fraud amounted to a billion or more dollars. Despite publicity, including a segment on the television news show *60 Minutes*, the government, insurers, physicians, and the public, were never adequately educated. The result: some waste continues.

The laboratory industry, however, educated itself. Industry publications discussed at length the theory of the fraud and whether "safe harbor" regulations offered protection from prosecution. Ironically, the education efforts and the widely disseminated laboratory industry publications became an important piece of evidence in proving the fraudulent intent by those laboratories, which continued the billings for the useless add-ons after publicized prosecutions.

On a smaller scale, a substantial number of providers facing criminal prosecution try the "bookkeeper defense." The bookkeeper defense refers to physicians claiming that their billings were improper because the bookkeeper was the one who chose the incorrect CPT code. An insurer who presents an effective education program regarding the dos and don'ts of billing will succeed in educating a substantial number of these bookkeepers. And an SIU which teaches physicians that they can go to jail if the bookkeeper errs will encourage physicians to educate their bookkeepers.

A persuasive way for the SIU to accomplish educational aims is delivering brief presentations at health-care seminars and educational programs. That's easier for larger providers, including hospitals and nursing home chains, which already undertake in-house education programs and welcome willing speakers.

In addition to deterring and preventing fraud, the education effort often reaps other benefits for the SIU. Speaking engagements may lead to tips on fraudulent schemes, or provide valuable evidence of intent when the educational effort is ignored in favor of the higher reimbursement rate.

Watching peers have to fork over big dollars to repay what they stole has, as already said, a powerful deterrent effect. But the mere single-damages recovery of money obtained unethically or illegally does little to deter a provider or his peers from thievery. The provider who is forced to repay only 70% of the money he stole has an incentive to renew his efforts as soon as the audit is concluded. Thus, an SIU whose primary aim is to recover stolen funds will often be faced with the task of recovering money for the same schemes, and even from the same providers, over and over again.

The situation is exacerbated by the litigious provider who forces the case to the brink of trial before settling for an amount that is substantially less than the SIU case has identified as overpaid. The insurer incurs substantial costs in preparing its case for trial, and fails to recover even the amounts it has paid out in connection with fraudulent and abusive claims. In order to avoid this losing proposition, the SIU must have a proverbial big stick to wield to place the provider in a worse position than if he had not committed the fraud. Jail is unquestionably the biggest stick available, so the SIU should strive to make sure more blatant frauds are prosecuted criminally.

The second biggest stick is a civil or administrative remedy involving large money penalties. With double or trebled damages and a per-claim fine, the potential award can practically approach satisfying the national debt. At the federal level, the Civil Monetary Penalties Law provides for double damages, plus up to $10,000 per false claim. The federal False Claims Act provides for trebled damages and up to $10,000 per false claim. Thus, the potential liability for nationwide fraud schemes can easily reach millions of dollars.

Another tool which has been used successfully by private insurers is the civil Racketeer Influenced and Corrupt Organizations Act (RICO). RICO provides for multiple damages and attorneys' fees in the event of a successful civil prosecution. Like a successful criminal prosecution, publicity regarding a crippling financial award educates the public about the existence of the SIU and dissuades other providers from fraudulent conduct.

CHAPTER 6

Marketing the SIU Inside And Outside Your Health Plan

Special investigations units (SIUs) must be marketed both inside the organization and beyond. Internal marketing efforts, launched with fraud awareness training, have begun to make the employees aware of the problem and what the insurer or managed care plan is doing to try and control it. While it's important to focus training on operations staff — such as claims processors, customer service staff, and claims coders — employees within the administrative function of the company also need to learn about the SIU.

Here are suggestions for getting the word to everyone about the SIU:

- Publish an article in any company newsletter. The article should include a definition of fraud; directions on how to make a referral; statistics on the prevalence of fraud; the phone extensions of the fraud control unit director and staff members; and the number of the fraud-reporting hotline, if you plan to have one.
- Introduce the SIU at management meetings.
- Institute a corporate anti-fraud policy that outlines the goals and objectives of the SIU.
- Integrate fraud awareness training into new-employee orientation.
- Develop employee incentive programs for those who refer cases to the SIU.

It's also critical to get to know, and build positive relationships with, individuals that you will need support from to get the SIU's job done. These include information systems staff, microfilm staff, and claims staff.

Hopefully, most employees will perceive these ideas as favorable, which will ultimately help garner upper management's support.

Getting the support and respect of upper management is critical to the success of any SIU. With their endorsement, you will be able to start and expand the unit. The SIU has to have backing because its effectiveness depends on the assistance of many other departments in the company. Profound support from above will help get your requests moved up the priority ladder.

How do you go about gaining the support and respect of upper management? The first step is to develop a fraudfighting plan. This plan will formulate ideas previously mentioned in this book, and it would incorporate other areas, such as the plan for workflow, case management, SIU policies and procedures, monthly reporting of statistics, and standards expected of SIU personnel.

This manual can be used to educate upper management about your function and to train SIU staff. The manual also can be submitted to the state agency that regulates fraud control units.

When developing the manual to educate upper management, present it as an executive summary of what the SIU is doing, how it's being done and why. The manual should be comprehensive and be approved by upper management before distribution.

The following is a sample table of contents that you might use in your fraud manual:

I. Administration
- A. Purpose
- B. Philosophy
- C. Summary of Job Titles
- D. Staffing Plan
- E. Space Plan
- F. Marketing Plan
- G. Monthly Reports
- H. Statistics
- I. Internal and SIU Policies

II. Investigation
- A. Definition of Fraud
- B. Work Flow
- C. Case Management
- D. Investigative Techniques
- E. Investigative Traps
- F. Report Writing

III. Post Investigation
- A. Decisions
- B. Closing the case
- C. Working with Law Enforcement

D. Responsibilities after case is closed
E. Standards

Another key method of building support is through statistics, which is proof positive that the SIU is a good return on the company's investment. Statistics can be a continuing reminder of the unit's value. The trap with statistics, though, is compiling an abundance of them can take up too much time. The trick: identify the areas that tell the most about your unit.

Here are examples of areas where statistics have the most compelling story to tell about the SIU:

- Number of open and closed cases: These numbers will represent how much work there is for the unit and how much work the unit is doing. You will also be able to show trends, such as the correlation between unit growth and caseload growth. Or you can show that there's a need for more staff because the backlog of cases is overwhelming.
- Number of cases, defined by case type: It may be important to show who the majority of the alleged perpetrators are, such as the proportion of abusive providers vs. subscribers. This may also help you in deciding where you need to focus your attentions and what type of people you need to hire.
- How many dollars were paid out in fraud: This figure is important because it will show how pervasive the problem is at your specific organization and will justify the need for the unit.
- How many fraud dollars were recovered and how many dollars were saved: There is a difference between recovering money and saving it. A recovery is any money that had been stolen from the insurer and was gotten back. Savings refers to money the SIU stopped from being paid out, by, for example, catching onto a scheme before it progressed very far. Savings is the more important figure, because any money that is saved is a guaranteed 100% return, while recoveries may be a fraction of the total amount of money lost in a scheme. Regardless, these figures will be a reminder of the savings your unit is making for the company and is the justification your unit needs for existence and expansion.
- Number of referrals made to the unit and the source of the referrals.
- Number of referrals made by the unit and where they are going.

These numbers should be compiled monthly, quarterly, year-to-date and annually.

In addition to building internal support, SIUs need the endorsement of outside segments of the health care and law enforcement communities. This includes providers, provider groups, members of law enforcement, state insurance departments, other carriers, and other interested parties, such as shareholders.

To reach these audiences, try:

- Issuing educational material within correspondence to providers, groups and members to inform them that you have started a fraud unit and to outline the unit's objectives.
- Publicizing the hotline in general mailings and printing the hotline number on statements to members or providers.
- Incorporating the unit into sales pitches or marketing plans and publicizing successful cases through the print media.
- Meeting regularly with law enforcement, state regulatory agencies and other health plans to inform them of your entrance into the anti-fraud arena.
- Joining, on a corporate or individual basis, any organizations relevant to health care fraud, becoming an active participant, and attending their meetings.

CHAPTER 7

Information Technology

As we move into the information age, it is vital that insurers have at least the same capabilities as health care providers. This means insurers must not only have the ability to process claims quickly and accurately, but must have sufficient ability to cross-check both providers' and ancillary services against historical data and against suspected patterns already programmed into the system. Each insurer should be able to duplicate the provider-based Surveillance and Utilization Review Subsystem utilizing existing technology (see Chapter 1).

In addition to this, however, an excellent fraud detection system should also be recipient-based and able to assure that services paid to one provider on behalf of a patient on a given date are not duplicated on that same date to another provider. Such a system will enable the immediate detection of claims submitted for duplicate services by either the same provider or different providers.

A sophisticated system will also be able to detect those instances in which the stated diagnosis on a submitted claim does not correspond with the services provided. A child, for example, being treated for an injured knee probably doesn't need diagnostic hearing services. Likewise, a nursing home-bound patient diagnosed as suffering from senile dementia probably won't benefit from office-based psychoanalysis from a mental health provider.

A sophisticated information technology system can cross-check the very nature of the patient against the types of services rendered. For example, sophisticated technology is able to record the date of a patient's death and automatically disallow all claims after that death. In addition, there are many types of health care services which are appropriate only for certain age groups. Perhaps an extreme example involves elderly patients on whose behalf family planning or maternity care is billed. Children under the age of five are the unlikely recipients of mental health services. It is highly unlikely that all members of the same family have the same diagnosis, receive the same blood test, and are treated with the same drug. Such an occurrence is far more likely to signal a health care provider has submitted false claims on behalf of one or all members of that family in an attempt to increase reimbursement.

The special investigations unit (SIU) cannot investigate a case without adequate access to data. One of the most important roles a new SIU will play is making sure that it opens the doors to get the information needed within the participating provider network, as well as at other agencies.

It is obvious that the SIU must have access to paid claims data submitted to the company, and that it must have contractual or other legal means of getting access to patient records maintained by the participating practitioners.

The task of getting adequate access to data is somewhat more challenging in a managed care setting, where the responsibility for providing services may be passed onto a network of health care practitioners which has only a minimal contractual relationship with the company. These providers may resist the requirement to open their data banks to the company for audit purposes, particularly where they have merged their records with those of non-company patients who are entitled to privacy. In addition, even if the electronic data is produced for the company, it may be in a different format and largely unusable by the SIU.

Moreover, when physicians are paid on a capitated basis, documentation is not a prerequisite for payment. Physicians may succumb to the temptation to reduce their record-keeping requirements and maintain fewer bits of evidence that a visit occurred. If the managed care plan does not have strict documentation maintenance requirements and holes in the records result, and the SIU isn't guaranteed access to data that does exist, the SIU will be hampered in its investigations of the appropriateness of out-of network referrals, adequacy of patient care (underutilization), kickbacks, and other frauds inherent to the managed care delivery system.

The SIU should be prepared to address the increased use of electronic media for medical records and physician orders, bringing with it the attendant need of the SIU to understand the potential for forgery and alteration of such a record. The electronic record keeping systems, if properly established, will be more secure and less subject to manipulation than their paper predecessors. Conversely, if a provider is able to manipulate the records, it will be more difficult to detect, correct and prosecute fraud. Present federal rules and regulations for computerized records of physician orders and recordkeeping are woefully inadequate, and the insurer which allows its practitioners to abandon paper documents should adopt additional electronic safeguards.

Without question, properly trained and dedicated agents are the most effective and expensive SIU asset against fraud. In turn, the agents' greatest tool will be computer hardware and software that are sophisticated and versatile enough to analyze, organize and compare the claims data for providers and beneficiaries. The SIU should purchase sufficient computer hardware and be prepared to upgrade the hardware every few years. SIU agents who do a lot of work in the providers' offices should be equipped with laptop computers.

Software selection is also important. Although the software itself is seldom a major expense, it can be costly to train SIU personnel to use it effectively. The SIU should compare database programs, selecting one that can move data fast and quickly organize and reorganize billings without cannibalizing time or memory. If the SIU has contractual or legal (e.g., search and seizure) access to download a provider's claims data in connection with an audit, the SIU should provide for mirror-image copying, safe storage, and a separate computer on which to store the claims data pending use at trial.

Increasingly sophisticated computer tools are available to store and maintain evidence. In a recent five-month-long health care fraud case in San Diego, California, claims and other documents were scanned and bar coded, and the image maintained in a computer. Throughout the trial, whenever a document was discussed, the operator keyed in the document number or bar code, and an image of that document was instantaneously projected on a screen for the benefit of the jury.

Other tools used by the SIU will depend upon the unit's goals and legal restrictions. Law enforcement units may legally employ surveillance techniques that SIUs are not allowed to use, thus making the SIU's investment in electronic "spy" equipment superfluous. The SIU's best equipment, regardless of technological advances, will always be a trained and willing worker with an agile mind.

CHAPTER 8

Preparing Cases

There are a number of ways for a special investigations unit (SIU) to identify fraudulent providers within its participating provider population. The most obvious ways include beneficiary complaints, comparisons of billing patterns between similar providers, and audits. Selected targeting mechanisms will, in large part, depend upon the size of the insurer, the number and diversity of its participating providers, and the geographical area covered by the SIU.

Increasingly, insurers are contracting with national health provider chains. In the past decade, ownership of pharmacy, laboratory, nursing home, mental health, durable medical equipment, and other providers has become consolidated through mergers and acquisitions. Hence, SIUs that unmask fraud schemes, such as kickbacks for referrals or deceptive marketing of laboratory tests, are likely to face a huge corporate provider with unlimited litigation resources and a nationwide motive for avoiding conviction or judgment.

These multi-jurisdictional providers may be quick to settle the case with a promise of non-disclosure in order to prevent publicity about the scheme and potential queries by other insurers. Non-disclosure agreements in settlements are routinely requested by providers and granted by SIUs eager to settle. But the practice perpetuates fraud by making it harder for insurers to share information on bad practices and errant providers. SIUs should consider adopting a policy against entering such agreements.

Before concluding that it cannot individually take on a Goliath-sized provider, the SIU should query whether there are similar actions by other insurers and governmental entities which the SIU could join.

Local providers who double bill, bill for non-existent patients, upcode, or perform unnecessary diagnostic procedures are commonly uncovered by complaints and an in-house audit program. Because these cases will be the SIU's bread and butter, attempts should be made to develop sources for referrals and liaisons with other insurers used by the providers in question, and to maintain good in-house access to information on past claims and provider education attempts.

With the possible exception of fake 'accident' victims and drug addicts, the cost of beneficiary fraud pales in comparison with the cost of provider fraud. Since beneficiary fraud prosecutions involve different methods of investigation and prosecution, the SIU that decides to prosecute beneficiary fraud should consider separate training and standards for the investigators assigned to handle this aspect of its work.

To prove a case of *criminal* fraud, it is necessary to show that the provider had criminal intent and used deception to take money to which it was not entitled. This is a difficult burden to prove. Anyone who has witnessed recent notorious trials can attest that the American jury system can be somewhat arbitrary and certainly very fluid. One easy test is to ask otherwise neutral persons the following question: Should the particular health care provider go to jail for his or her conduct? If the answer is no, it means a prosecutor will have a very difficult time establishing to a jury that the acts in question constitute criminal fraud.

It is vital to remember as we pursue these types of investigations that the health care field is one of the more heavily regulated professions in our society today. Investigators and prosecutors in this field repeatedly hear perpetrators contend that ignorance of arcane and often obtuse rules or overworked billing clerks are to blame for "errors."

To rebut such an "ignorance" or "bookkeeper" defense, the best proof of criminal intent arises from the provider's attempt to conceal the crime. For example, a provider may receive a subpoena from a law enforcement authority or a written request from an insurance company to provide records supporting his billing practices. If those records are later proved to be altered in a substantial way in an effort to mask the suspect billing pattern, this constitutes excellent proof that the provider not only committed a fraud, but knew that he committed a fraud and was attempting to conceal it. Obviously, such a provider would be hard-pressed to later claim that he did not understand the rules, or to blame his employees.

Medicare investigators in Florida, for example, found instances in which a particular health care provider was offering patients money if these patients would submit their unopened explanation-of-benefits letters to the provider. Of course, it later developed that the provider was billing for excessive numbers of services on behalf of these patients, all of which would have been discovered had the patients opened their letters and reviewed the statement. Nevertheless, by giving patients money, the provider supplied investigators with ample proof that he knew that the activities which he was undertaking were fraudulent and required concealment.

In addition to providing excellent evidence of the providers' intent, such concealment may be a crime in and of itself. Any effort to conceal or alter records once they have been properly subpoenaed by a criminal authority can result in obstruction of justice charges. Most federal and state judges view a charge of obstruction of justice as a direct threat against the judicial authority of the court system and will likely impose a sentence of incarceration in the event a successful case is proved.

Other excellent evidence of concealment may arise if the provider instructs her personnel to fabricate excuses for why the billing occurred, or otherwise instructs them to mislead investigators in their efforts to determine the truth. A provider who instructs her staff to lie to investigators would find it difficult to later assert her innocence of the underlying billing fraud.

Another excellent piece of evidence in this regard arises from instances in which providers repeatedly ignore warnings from insurers that their billing method is improper. In fact, juries often like to see some attempt on the part of the insurer to find an amicable resolution to the matter before referring it for prosecution. Therefore, such letters in which providers are warned to correct their billing patterns are often appropriate. Nevertheless, providers ignoring those warnings furnish solid evidence they knew what they were doing and that it was wrong.

Other cases that can be proven with little or no leg work typically involve good information technology or witnesses with first-hand knowledge. Examples in this area may include bills submitted on days when the provider was not open for business or, better yet, was out of town. Prosecutors have succeeded against physicians who bill for services on dates when it is later established the physician was in distant locales. Most juries are offended by such conduct and will decide against the provider. In this regard, the physician's *unaltered* appointment book is a vital piece of evidence. Credit card receipts, airline tickets, U.S. Customs information, American Automobile Association information, car rental agency paperwork, and any number of sources can provide useful information in this regard.

Once it can be established to a jury that a physician billing for the delivery of a baby was, in fact, at a distant medical conference at the time of that alleged delivery, little sympathy will remain for the provider.

Earlier, reference was made to the fact that a good investigator must determine whether the physician has the necessary equipment and personnel to render the services for which he or she bills. Once again, if it can be established at trial that a health care provider is billing for laboratory tests, complicated medical services, or an inordinate volume of services not possible to have been performed given the circumstances, courts will likely find that a fraud was perpetrated and will not accept the defense of "mistake."

Evidence that the health care provider double-billed for services already rendered by that provider or others can also be a good indicator of fraud. Examples include a dentist who bills for extracting the same tooth twice or for a tooth previously extracted by another provider; a physician who bills for rendering identical medical tests on successive dates; or an obstetrician who bills for delivering a baby within one or two months of when he submitted another bill for the delivery by the same mother.

SIU Staff Needs to Understand Laws

The first step in preparing a case for trial is to understand the elements of the crime to be charged. The most egregious fraud in the company's history is not a good case if you cannot locate a statute prohibiting the conduct, or if the conduct occurred outside the statute of limitations. Key SIU staff must, therefore, be familiar with the available criminal statutory alternatives — both state and federal — which are relevant to the crimes under investigation.

A working knowledge of the elements of the crime is important to gathering evidence for the investigation, as well as to selecting the forum in which it will be prosecuted. Statutes relating to health care may be as simple as theft, false claims, or prohibitions against altering medical records, or as complex as anti-kickback laws or self-referral bans. Pay attention to the statute of limitations which, for many state crimes, may be as little as one year.

Also important to investigating health care fraud is an understanding of the potential civil and administrative remedies, and how the SIU can make use of them. The federal government and some states have powerful civil false claims statutes that require a lower standard of proof, yet provide for huge monetary recoveries and potential exclusion from the federally funded health care programs.

Putting together a good fraud case is of little use if you cannot convince a prosecutor to charge the crime. The SIU must explore the available options for criminal, civil, and administrative prosecutions, and develop a forum in which its cases will be prosecuted. The manner in which the case is prepared and presented will depend upon the available prosecutorial resources. It is critical for the SIU to understand its options and limitations before investing the time and effort in preparing a case for trial, as the manner in which the case is developed is often dictated by the statutes and practices of the prosecuting attorneys.

In most states, SIUs will have four avenues leading to court: federal, state, local, and in-house civil fraud prosecutions.

Federal: The U.S. attorneys' offices have broad jurisdiction to prosecute fraud against Medicare, Medicaid and other federal health plans. The U.S. attorneys also can prosecute fraud against private insurers under the broad authority to prosecute wire and mail frauds. For the first time, thanks to the new insurance reform law, legal recourse exists against health fraud perpetrators under a new federal crime of health fraud (see Chapter 11). The law also beefed up the penalties that can be assessed for Medicare and Medicaid fraud. These statutes are broad, their statutes of limitations generally expansive, and the quality of the prosecutors and judges are generally good. If they accept a case for trial, the attorneys will devote the necessary time and effort to increase the odds of a successful outcome.

On the other hand, federal prosecutors have responsibility for prosecuting many crimes other than health fraud, and have limited resources. Busier offices have minimum loss and other standards, and may not accept a viable fraud case that does not meet those standards. Few offices would hesitate to discuss their criteria for accepting a case from an SIU that wants to refer matters for criminal disposition.

State: Most states have Medicaid fraud control units, which will be eager to prosecute a well-developed case that involves harm to the Medicaid program, and will be willing to tack on counts relating to fraud against a private insurer so your SIU can get a piece of the action. The units have immense health care prosecutorial experience because they are required by law to devote their resources solely to the prosecution of health care matters. Since unscrupulous providers often fail to discriminate when it comes to defrauding insurers, the SIU should be on the lookout for fraud having a nexus to the Medicaid program. The Medicaid fraud control units prosecute in state courts, using state statutes.

Even if there is no Medicaid nexus, many states have specialized white-collar criminal prosecution units in the state attorneys general offices. These units generally accept high-profile and complicated matters for trial, and are usually willing to devote the time and resources necessary to win the case.

Local: Local district attorneys have jurisdiction over the prosecution of most criminal matters, from shoplifting to murder. The offices often have specialized units to handle complex financial crimes, but will invariably have heavier dockets and fewer resources than state or federal agencies. The SIU's success in getting a local district attorney to take a case and aggressively prosecute it will depend upon the particular talents and priorities of the district attorney's office and the strength of the SIU liaison with that office.

***In-house*:** Handling the prosecution of fraud cases in-house is a viable alternative for larger SIUs. The prosecution of a civil fraud or racketeering allegation is manpower-intensive and expensive, but can lead to huge, well-publicized verdicts in favor of the SIU. And, though jail is not an option, the errant provider will be harshly punished by the punitive award and, in many states, the attendant revocation or suspension of a medical license. Key to the decision to litigate such a case in-house is the depth of the SIU litigation team and the jury appeal of the particular case.

Finally, the SIU should be aware of administrative agencies and their work. Licensing and certifying agencies which deal with public safety issues may be willing to investigate quality assurance violations. Although their investigation may not yield a monetary recovery or criminal statistic, these agencies may revoke or suspend the license of a provider having bad claims as the result of poor quality care. Obviously, if the provider has no license, he or she cannot continue to submit claims for inadequate services.

There is an important caveat to pursuing fraud cases: Every possibility must be explored that "fraudulent billing" was not actually a mistake on the part of the provider. Computer glitches, sloppy staff work, or other less nefarious errors can sometimes explain these billing irregularities and must be fully explored by the insurers or those investigating allegations of fraud. Providers may successfully use billing irregularities as a defense, after the insurer will have expended considerable time and resources investigating potential fraud. It is always wise to explore these potential defenses at the inception of the investigation to assure that you are dealing with true fraudulent billing patterns and not just a mistake on the part of the provider.

CHAPTER 9

Referring Cases Outside Your Organization

Whenever there is well-grounded suspicion of criminal fraud, you should almost always refer a suspected fraud case to an appropriate authority. From the standpoint of the insurer, there is no legal risk posed by the referral unless it is frivolous or solely in retribution against the provider for reasons unrelated to criminal activity. For example, if an insurer has had difficult relations with the provider, and is referring the case solely to "get even," such a referral could subject the insurer to charges of frivolous prosecution and result in a lawsuit against the insurer by the provider. Nevertheless, frivolous referrals have been exceedingly rare and there is no legal exposure for an insurer making a factually-grounded referral to a prosecuting authority.

From the standpoint of law enforcement professionals, a potentially powerful criminal case against a provider could be harmed if an untrained investigator has contact with that provider. If law enforcement personnel are involved early in the investigatory process, it may be possible for them to conduct an undercover investigation before the provider learns he or she is suspected of fraud.

Further, any representations made by the insurer to the provider may later prove detrimental to a criminal investigation. These representations may include false assurances that the provider has done nothing of concern, conflicting advice about the proper billing code to use, or affirmative advice to a provider on methods to circumvent seemingly innocuous regulations of the insurer. All of these representations can later be used by a provider to establish complicity on the part of the insurer's staff, causing a jury to look less harshly on the provider's misconduct.

Another area of potential concern for prosecutors is the possibility that the insurance investigator may become the *de facto* agent of the law enforcement agency in situations where the insurance investigator takes instructions from the prosecutor, leading to questions of evidence integrity and authority. Thus, once a case is referred by the insurer, the investigative role of the insurer will be limited.

Demands Heavy on Insurers Who Refer Cases

If a criminal or civil prosecution is pursued by government authorities, the claims of the insurer can be included in the amount demanded as restitution, and the insurer will recover that amount in the event of successful litigation. It is important to recognize, however, that this requires a commitment to assist the law enforcement agency or the prosecuting authority in preparing the case for trial. The insurer or managed care plan's staff time may be needed in order to assist prosecutors with claims review or testimony about facts relevant to the prosecution. These investigations and prosecutions are frequently time consuming and, depending on the nature of the prosecution, can take several years. Insurers may find it easier and quicker to attempt recovery of this money on their own without referring the matter to a prosecuting authority.

Indeed, the health care provider under suspicion may be the first to request a private settlement because his or her fear of criminal prosecution and its attendant consequences are immense. Insurers opting to pursue their own civil remedies, though, must expend considerable legal fees to pursue an appropriate legal action, and they forego the substantial deterrence effect a prosecution can have on other providers in the field.

In addition, patients aware of actions against providers for abusive activities will become more concerned about the nature of their care and have greater regard for their insurers' willingness to tackle fraud. Therefore, they will more likely report to their insurers activity which they deem suspicious. In sum, the cost savings and intangible benefits which result from referring cases for criminal prosecution, though difficult to quantify, often far exceed that which is recovered by insurers settling with providers behind closed doors.

There is no legal duty imposed on providers to refer a case to law enforcement except in those cases with pharmaceutical or antitrust implications. However, there are several legal issues which make referrals advisable.

For example, the Civil Monetary Penalties Law imposes liability on providers who *knew or should have known* of false billing. For example, the acts of a managed care employee can result in liability imposed against the entire managed care plan if the provider reasonably should have known of those acts. A physician who is committing fraud blatantly while employed by a managed care plan can subject the entire managed care plan to civil monetary penalties, which can be extensive and also result in the exclusion of the plan from government insurance programs, such as Medicare and Medicaid.

There are additional incentives for health care providers, such as managed care plans, to voluntarily assist in ferreting out fraud within their plans. Federal sentencing guidelines, for example, provide for lesser sentences against those providers who voluntarily assist in the investigation and prosecution of fraud. Also, the HHS office of inspector general's voluntary disclosure program, which is still in its pilot stage, may permit health care providers to escape criminal sanctions if a disclosure is made to law enforcement or Department of Health and Human Services' investigators before the government learns of actual fraudulent activity.

For example, a managed care plan which notices that its employees have committed fraud against Medicare or Medicaid may voluntarily disclose that information to the Department of Health and Human Services and escape criminal prosecution, assuming that HHS had not already learned of this scheme.

'Whistleblowers' Have Financial Incentives to Expose Fraud

The relatively new phenomena of litigation sparked by the "qui tam" provisions of the False Claims Act has caused many health care providers to undertake voluntary disclosure in order to minimize the risk posed by employees and others who may reporting misdeeds to federal authorities as whistleblowers.

Under the false claims law, whistleblowers have immense financial incentives to reveal to government investigators any fraud committed by health care providers against a government insurance plan. Federal law permits such whistleblowers to file a lawsuit against the health care provider on behalf of the United States, seeking to recover the amounts fraudulently obtained by the provider. If successful, the whistleblower will obtain a percentage of the amounts recovered on behalf of the government.

In addition, the United States Department of Justice has the opportunity to take over the whistleblower's lawsuit and bring to bear the various resources of the federal government in litigating against the health care provider.

The qui tam provision deserves note for two reasons. First, the cases are widely publicized when settled or unsealed, and the special investigations unit (SIU) can then determine if it has been the target of similar fraud by the provider. Secondly, an aggressive and innovative SIU may become a whistleblower if it has personal knowledge of a fraud against a governmental interest that is covered by a qui tam statute.

There have been several recent national false claims cases which originated with a whistleblower, as plaintiff, filing a lawsuit against a former employer or, in one case, competitor about whom the litigant had knowledge of fraud. The result can be very lucrative for the whistleblower. Such lawsuits can also provide a substantial incentive on the part of health care plans to maintain great vigilance in determining whether any of their employees are committing acts against the federal government which could result in a large monetary claim by the government.

Insurers, on the other hand, are under no obligation to refer cases for prosecution in which a health care provider may have stolen money from a private insurance company. However, private insurers which are publicly held may have a duty to stockholders to disclose losses and the cause of those losses. Failure to properly investigate and refer to the appropriate authority may constitute a breach of fiduciary duty to stockholders of the insurer.

As a result, many insurers have taken an increasingly aggressive stance in investigating fraud committed by health care providers and then referring to appropriate authorities the information that is obtained as a result of that investigation. As indicated earlier, health care fraud has garnered the attention of a variety of state and federal authorities, as well as private entities. All of these organizations can be valuable resources to anti-fraud efforts.

The National Health Care Anti-Fraud Association is a national, voluntary association which consists of private insurers, health care providers, regulatory authorities, and federal and state law enforcement personnel. It meets regularly to share information and learn new techniques in fraud detection (and methods of fraud commission). The assiciation also supports state and federal legislative initiatives to battle fraud.

The Department of Justice and United States attorneys in all 50 states have established health care fraud working groups which seek the input of private industry to enforcement and fraud prevention measures. Often they have quarterly meetings with private insurers in the health care field both to obtain their input and to determine whether there are health care providers meriting closer attention by federal investigative authorities.

The FBI is more active than ever in the area of health care fraud and is a working member of the National Health Care Anti-Fraud Association. Larger states have at least one agent detailed to health care fraud issues. These agents are working closely with Medicaid fraud control units, United States attorneys, and other federal investigative authorities such as agents of the Office of Inspector General, Health and Human Services, CHAMPUS investigators, and other federal agents whose task it is to protect federal funds flowing into the health care field.

And, as mentioned earlier, 48 states now have Medicaid fraud control units to investigate and prosecute Medicaid fraud. However, the federal government will grant authority to these units to investigate and prosecute private insurance fraud in the event that these claims are ancillary to claims of Medicaid fraud. In other words, if a provider has stolen money both from Medicaid and from a private insurance plan, the Medicaid fraud control unit can receive permission to prosecute claims on behalf of insurers against that provider. This permission has, to date, been liberally granted by the Office of Inspector General, Health and Human Services. (These units also will prosecute patient abuse and neglected committed by Medicaid providers).

Under a new initiative funded by the Justice Department's Bureau of Justice Assistance, the attorneys general of Wisconsin, Maryland and Minnesota are working closely with private health insurers and state and federal agencies to develop new ways to combat private health care fraud, including fraud in managed care.

CHAPTER 10

Managed Care Fraud

The advent of managed care plans and captitated payment structures create new challenges to policing efforts. Since the traditional scheme involving overutilization will not necessarily result in a provider's enrichment under a capitated system, a fundamental question arises: What is a scheme to defraud under managed care?

Some indications can be gleaned from the HHS inspector general's October 1996 advisory bulletin on Medicare HMO enrollees' rights. Though it is written for consumers, the bulletin is useful for the health care field because it indicates the kinds of practices the government will scrutinize and, perhaps, penalize in lawsuits, intermediate sanctions or even criminal prosecutions (see Appendix for full text of HMO advisory bulletin).

Here are some of the government's rules on managed care practices that, if violated, may become fodder for government punitive actions:

- HMOs must give prospective Medicare members complete, accurate information on the plan.
- All Medicare eligibles who want to sign up for the managed care plan must be enrolled, regardless of age or health status.
- HMOs can't try to stop members from dropping the plan, and must process disenrollment requests promptly.
- HMOs can't offer potential enrollees gifts or money to enroll, except for snacks and promotional items worth less than $10.
- HMOs can't avoid providing medically necessary care in a prompt way.
- HMOs can't demand that emergency care be provided only at their facilities.

Lack of Care Can Be Fraud

Generally, when it comes to managed care fraud, law enforcement authorities have taken the position that schemes don't have to result in actual monetary loss to the victim or necessarily involve actual money or property loss. Instead, such things as intangible rights may be at issue. The test is "uprightness and fundamental honesty" under the circumstances.

This is relevant as it relates to managed care plans in situations in which a managed care plan sets up a system where patients are not receiving the care for which the government is paying. In such instances, it is conceivable that the federal government will maintain at least a civil cause of action to recover money and to impose civil penalties. A scheme to defraud includes a breach of a fiduciary relationship in which one party entrusts confidence in another. This traditionally includes a doctor-patient relationship.

Other statutes under which managed care plans can be prosecuted include those proscribing false statements, which holds that "whoever, in any matter within jurisdiction of the department or agency of the United States, knowingly and willfully falsifies, conceals or covers up by any trick, scheme or artifice the material fact, or makes any false, fictional, or fraudulent statements or representations, or makes or uses any false reading document," will be liable for criminal penalties (18 U.S.C. §1001). Another federal false claims statute also makes it a crime to submit a false claim, or a false or fraudulent document in support of a claim, to the United States. Mail fraud statutes extend these provisions to any scheme or artifice to defraud or obtain money by means of false or fraudulent pretenses by using the mails.

As it relates to managed care plans, the government authorities are particularly concerned about the denial of services or the unavailability of services after a plan has successfully won a contract to provide such services. These cases will be proved by using representations made to beneficiaries (1) by the plan in its marketing tactics; (2) by treating physicians working for the plan; (3) by sales representatives and contractors; (4) by documents executed by the plan; or (5) by customer service representatives.

In the event of such an investigation, the HMO's internal records, including the utilization tracking system which the plan employs, will become evidence. Other evidence will include accounting and actuarial records, evidence of any threats, inducements, bonuses or recognition employed by the plan toward its employees or subcontractors, recorded measurements of "quality of outcomes," and sales and marketing materials.

Managed care plans must be wary of offering incentives to their sales representatives to enroll patients in their plans for fear that these sales representatives will abuse their authority and offer illegal inducements to patients for enrollment. Of particular concern to regulatory authorities is so-called cherrypicking, the practice of sales representatives dangling inducements to lure seemingly healthy patients to enroll in a managed care plan, while discouraging presumably less healthy patients from enrolling. Such practices on the part of sales representatives and managed care plans could result in prosecution under various anti-kickback statutes, both state and federal.

Several states have undertaken investigations and prosecutions of sales representatives working on behalf of managed care plans who register fictitious enrollees or offer inducements to enrollees to subscribe to a managed care plan. The state of Maryland, for example, recently prosecuted several sales representatives from four managed care plans who made false representations to Medicaid recipients about the benefits they'd receive, the potential for winning prizes for enrolling, and other incentives which caused Medicaid recipients to enroll in plans and thereby enriched those sales representatives working on a commission basis. Some states have recently considered legislation which would outlaw commission-based sales to their Medicaid populations.

Fraud Against Managed Care Plans

Given the competitive nature of the industry, managed care plans should also be concerned with fraud committed *against* their plans. High on this list will be prescription drug diversion by physicians, patients and pharmacists. Also included are false financial status reports by providers, the falsification of quality reporting and records, employee health care providers who directly solicit payments from enrollees for covered services, kickbacks to managed care officials by physicians or other health care providers in order to join or remain in the network, and misrepresentations made by providers about secondary payers.

Of course, at the inception, a managed care plan must be very careful to curtail the possibility of fraud. Ways to accomplish this include:

- Establishing a compliance program reasonably capable of reducing the prospect of criminal conduct.

- Designating a responsible officer to oversee compliance.
- Exercising care not to delegate discretionary authority to persons with a propensity toward crime.
- Communicating compliance standards effectively to employees through training programs and publications.
- Taking reasonable steps to achieve compliance with those standards by implementing extensive monitoring, auditing and reporting systems; and
- Enforcing the standards by disciplining violators and taking reasonable steps to avoid recurrence of such acts.

Managed care plans must be extra vigilant when developing physician compensation arrangements. In the past, one of the primary concerns of government authorities has been to avoid overutilization. Specifically, any financial incentives which would cause a physician to order medical services over and above those deemed medically necessary have drawn the strict scrutiny of enforcement agencies. Under a capitated system, this concern has shifted to underutilization, which is the failure to render necessary care.

Use Experts to Review Physician Contracts

Several statutes have been enacted to address this concern, most notably 42 U.S.C. §1395mm(I)(a). It prohibits HMOs from operating physician incentive plans in such a way as to hamper the provision of medically necessary services to enrollees. Title 42, section 1320a-7a(b)(1) of the United States Code prohibits hospitals from making payments to physicians to induce them to reduce or limit services to Medicare and Medicaid patients.

This enforcement approach takes aim at a variety of financial relationships, including: (1) contracts with physicians that allegedly compromise physician objectivity regarding choice of provider; (2) promotional activities by pharmaceutical companies that encourage physicians to recommend certain products over others; (3) HMO or hospital management contracts that allegedly interfere with physicians' judgments regarding admissions, referrals, lengths of stay, and treatment protocols; and (4) clinical laboratory deals which influence physician objectivity with respect to the ordering of lab tests.

When establishing a relationship with a physician, a managed care plan must be very careful to assure that the physician is not paid "too much" so to appear as if the plan is paying for physician referrals. On the other hand, if a physician is paid too little, the government may assume the reverse: that the physician is looking for plan referrals. This is a complex regulatory field, so a managed care plan should seek the advice of competent counsel before entering into any compensation arrangements with a physician. The numerous federal regulations in this area, including safe harbors to the Medicare anti-kickback law, require an extensive knowledge of the relevant laws and should not be left to chance or cursory examination.

One state, Arizona, has instituted a reporting requirement imposed on managed care providers requiring that any incident of potential fraud and abuse which has occurred must be reported by the managed care plan to the state agency entrusted with investigations. In fact, Arizona law says that the failure of a managed care provider to report these episodes could lead to suspension of the state contract and significant money penalties (*Arizona Health Care Cost Containment System Health Plans and Program Contractors: Policy for Prevention, Detection and Reporting of Fraud and Abuse,* pp. 901-903, 1995).

The state of Tennessee has instituted similar requirements on managed care providers.

The areas of fraud which regulators have focused on here include (1) soliciting, offering and receiving kickbacks, bribes or rebates; (2) violating agreements, such as between providers and the plan, or the plan and the state; (3) entering false or misleading information on cost reports; and (4) enrolling members by using false information.

Probably the most difficult cases to investigate are those which question the medical necessity of the services rendered. To investigate such cases, it is critical that the investigators be medically trained, preferably in the field or in the specialty of the provider. Many law enforcement agencies in this area have learned that it is necessary to use medical experts who treat the same or similar health populations as those of the provider under investigation.

If at all possible, it is wise to avoid "ivory tower experts," whose sole experience in a particular area may be in academia or with patient populations demographically different from those of the provider under investigation.

Standards of treatment throughout the nation vary widely, even within the same specialty fields, and it is important that any investigation address this discrepancy. It is altogether likely that a health care provider treating an underprivileged or poor population from an inner city exercises far different standards of care than those within rural areas or more affluent neighborhoods. While one can reasonably debate the social policy attendant to such discrepancies of care, the bottom line for an insurer or other investigator is far more practical: whether the provider committed fraud or merely adhered to the standards of the particular practice within that area. Only those health care providers practicing within that area can give the investigator a reasonable guidepost to that standard of care.

CHAPTER 11

New Challenges Private Insurers Face In Fighting Health Fraud

By Kirk J. Nahra*

As noted, the private sector plays a key part in fighting health care fraud. Its motivation stems from the fact that private payers cover 56% of the nation's total health care bill — with insurers paying 37% and consumers paying 19%.

Moreover, experience clearly shows that the health care provider who is defrauding Medicare, Medicaid, CHAMPUS (the Civilian Health and Medical Program of the Uniformed Services) or other government programs in all likelihood is also defrauding private payers, and vice versa. If one private payer is ripped off, typically multiple payers are victimized.

Because of the scope of the problem, the private sector in recent years has redoubled its anti-fraud efforts, both as individual companies and collectively.

Unfortunately, however, some potential stumbling blocks to private-payer fraudfighting may have been constructed — including parts of the Health Insurance Portability and Accountability Act, enacted in August 1996. The new law's provisions beef up fraud enforcement and provide for more guidance on whether specific business dealings implicate health fraud laws.

But the law also does little to help private-payer fraudbusting and may in fact interfere with public-private cooperation against fraud. Other complications include the changing financial incen-

---

*This chapter was written by Kirk J. Nahra, with Wiley, Rein & Fielding in Washington, D.C. It first appeared as a supplement to *Healthcare Business & Legal Strategies*, a newsletter published by AIS.

tives under managed care and the advent of electronic data interchange, which are addressed later in this chapter.

Public, Private Sectors Join Forces

The biggest group combating health care fraud is the National Health Care Anti-Fraud Association, established to combine the anti-fraud efforts of private sector health care payers with those of the public sector agencies responsible for investigating and prosecuting health care fraud.

The cooperative, issue-based association's member organizations account for most of the private and public health insurance benefits paid in the United States. Its objective is to improve the private and public sectors' ability to detect, investigate, prosecute both civilly and criminally, and, ultimately, prevent health care fraud.

Private insurers as well are becoming increasingly active in pursuing fraud. At the law enforcement level, insurers and other private payers routinely cooperate with law enforcement officials in investigating and prosecuting health care fraud.

On the civil side, a number of major lawsuits have been brought against providers, either by individual companies or by groups of insurers.

As private payers become more aggressive about fighting fraud, what are the hot topics for the next few years?

Reform Offers Mixed Support

The anti-fraud provisions of the Health Insurance Portability and Accountability Act of 1996, also known as the Kennedy-Kassebaum law, raise a number of new issues for private payers.

The law increases the federal government's ability to investigate and prosecute health care fraud. Overall, it should significantly boost the government's fight against health fraud, but the effect on private payers is not at all clear.

The basic provisions: The legislation creates a coordinated anti-fraud program under the direction of the U.S. Health and Human Services' inspector general and the attorney general, to be established by Jan. 1. This program will coordinate, oversee and direct state and federal health care fraud enforcement.

The law also creates a trust fund for implementation of the anti-fraud program. The trust fund includes (1) money appropriated by Congress to provide a specified baseline for the financing of health care fraud investigations; and (2) fines and penalties obtained from the prosecution of health care criminals.

On the criminal front, the law includes important new criminal provisions, making health care fraud a crime, expanding asset forfeiture for those crimes, increasing the government's ability to use injunctive relief to freeze illegally obtained assets, and establishing a broad crime of false statements. All of those new crimes apply to both public and private sector fraud.

The Kennedy-Kassebaum law also expands substantially numerous administrative and civil sanctions and extends them to a broader range of federal health care programs.

Little Private Gain from Most Provisions

Despite the benefits to law enforcement, the legislation does little to help private parties protect themselves from fraud.

The private sector is not ignored, as the bill includes some all-payer provisions, meaning perpetrators can be prosecuted for fraud against either public or private payers.

Most notably, the law creates a crime of health care fraud, which makes illegal any efforts to defraud any health care payer, no matter how the fraud is conducted. That statute will fill in some existing gaps in the statutory scheme and provide a useful criminal enforcement tool.

There is a significant omission, however. Because the crime is not included as a "predicate act" under the Racketeer Influenced and Corrupt Organizations, or RICO, statute, the new health fraud offense will have no substantial relevance to civil RICO cases. Accordingly, the provision will have little impact for private payers, except in federal criminal prosecutions.

The law includes few other provisions that provide direct, consistent benefits to private payers.

Potential obligations for private payers: Moreover, there are a number of areas in which private payers have concerns about how administrative implementation of Kennedy-Kassebaum will affect the private fight against health care fraud.

For example, in developing the coordinated anti-fraud program, the HHS secretary and the attorney general are required to "consult with and arrange for the sharing of data with representatives of health plans." There is no more specificity on this obligation, nor discussion of the role of private payers in fighting health care fraud.

While recognizing the benefit of private sector anti-fraud activity, the program "guidelines" could unfairly burden private sector efforts if the guidelines require payers to furnish a lot of information.

The legislation also creates a database to maintain information on providers that have been sanctioned for health care fraud and abuse. But the database is limited to "final adverse actions," a phrase that excludes "settlements in which no findings of liability have been made" — leaving out most settlements.

The bill requires health plans and government agencies to report final adverse actions, although there are no penalties for failing to report information.

It's also unclear who has responsibility for reporting criminal cases tied to private health care dollars — the prosecutor, the private payer, or perhaps even multiple private payers affected by the same criminal behavior. The guidelines may require too much material from private payers.

Another potential burden is a new "administrative subpoena" structure that will make it easier for the government to subpoena private payer records concerning the payer's own investigations. The government may require cooperation from private payers where the government formerly relied on informal cooperation.

Potential risks to public-private cooperation: With these potential burdens and the increased ability of law enforcement to fight fraud in government programs, there is a concern that the law, if not properly implemented, could derail public-private cooperation on fraud investigations.

While the program recognizes that the sharing of investigative information facilitates the overall effort against health care fraud, the imbalances created by the law create some significant risks that such cooperation will be diminished.

The biggest concern is that the federal government will focus even more on fraud against public programs such as Medicare, and less on private sector claims. Moreover, public payer fraud recoveries may be added to the anti-fraud trust fund, creating additional incentives for law enforcement to pursue only fraud against public programs, and perhaps unfairly prejudicing private payer efforts to recover stolen money.

Additionally, the government can use its new legislative authority to control money that may be due private payers. Because the bill allows forfeitures for public and private fraud, the government can exercise control over what is lawfully private money.

The government can direct the distribution of forfeited money; all details about any distribution are unspecified, including who may make such claims or how amounts are to be determined.

The forfeiture provision may be combined with new injunctive relief provisions that would allow the U.S. attorney general to bring suit to stop anyone "committing or about to commit a federal health care offense," and could result in the freezing of assets that otherwise might be available to private claimants.

Adapting Fraudfighting to Managed Care

The Kennedy-Kassebaum law creates numerous theoretical issues for fraudfighting, providing a framework for the legislative and law enforcement agendas over the next few years. In more immediate terms, one of the critical challenges for health care fraud investigators is how to adapt a fee-for-service anti-fraud mentality to a managed care payment environment.

Managed care, in its various permutations, changes many of the motivations and opportunities that lead to health care fraud. The key is to analyze and understand how managed care affects the nature of fraud and the tools necessary for fighting fraud. Unfortunately, such differences have not been a focus of either the people involved in creating the business of managed care or most active fraud investigators.

Fee-for-service gives the unscrupulous provider the incentive to do more (or claim to do more) in order to bill more and, therefore, be paid more. Most of the prominent fraud cases to date have involved such fraud — billing for services not rendered, kickbacks to increase referrals, and upcoding.

As costs in fee-for-service medicine skyrocketed, health care payers developed various mechanisms to "manage" the care provided to insureds. All of the various approaches to "managing" care, whether through utilization review, HMOs, PPOs or otherwise, distribute financial risk and cost-control incentives to reduce overall health care expenditures.

Managed care business developments have led to a number of different ways for fraud to be perpetrated and, correspondingly, to be investigated and prosecuted. Managed care alters the fundamental nature of some frauds that dishonest providers can commit, and expands the opportunities for creative abuse of the health care financing system.

For example, when a provider is paid a fixed "capitation" payment for potentially unlimited treatment of a given patient, the incentive for the unscrupulous provider is to provide less care in return for that payment — to underserve the patient — because the cost of providing treatment reduces the provider's "profit" from the fixed payment.

In day-to-day patient dealings, fraud involving the deliberate underprovision of care might include inadequate treatment; "automatic" referral of sicker, and thus more costly, patients to providers outside the capitated network (perhaps in exchange for kickbacks from those outside providers); and the establishment of inconvenient service locations and appointment hours for managed care patients, designed to suppress patient traffic.

In general, the types of frauds that occur in a managed care setting will be more subtle and, perhaps, more difficult to detect. Accordingly, fraud investigators must bear in mind a number of key issues as health care businesses and law enforcers adapt their anti-fraud efforts:

(1) Fee-for-service will continue to be a part of our health care system. There are few pure managed care models in which every patient service is delivered on a prepaid or fixed-cost basis. Therefore, tried and true fraudfighting tenets will not be abandoned, and investigators must understand how integrated payment systems containing managed care and fee-for-service elements operate.

(2) In a managed care setting, the core of the fraud scheme may be more difficult to demonstrate, even when providers indisputably are capitalizing on weaknesses in the system. In a "billing for services not rendered" case, the fraudulent elements are not in doubt. If the physician or provider bills for something he or she did not do, there is no question that the behavior is both improper and criminal. In a managed care setting, however, it may be less clear that a provider who has taken a capitated fee for serving a patient population, and then makes it difficult for patients to receive services, has committed a criminal act.

As a result of these marketplace changes, the detection and investigation of fraud in managed care operations will place new and far greater demands on fraud investigators. There are dozens of payment options in operation in the marketplace, with new choices emerging each day. Investigators will need to develop a much more sophisticated understanding of the variety and complexity of contractual arrangements between managed care payers and providers to understand the weak links in their particular system.

Part of the task for fraud investigators will be to understand where best to attack the problem, including who has the best access to relevant information.

As managed care has developed, more and more hybrid organizations have emerged, combining provider and payer functions in single entities. Larger, centralized operations also have emerged to take advantage of volume cost savings and improved risk management and assessment. Such middlemen may become the best means of uncovering complex frauds. At the same time, the middleman operations may also be the mechanism for conducting fraud, causing a "fox guarding the chicken coop" problem.

Electronic Data Interchange Brings New Fraud Risks

The other key business issue confronting private payers involves the transition to electronic claims processing. With increasing speed, health care payers across the country are moving from a paper-based system to one that relies on electronic submission and payment of health care claims. The administrative simplification provisions of the Kennedy-Kassebaum reform law require Electronic Data Interchange (EDI) capability for all significant payers in a short time frame.

So far, fraud concerns have not been a focus of discussions of electronic data interchange. In other industries that have undertaken the conversion to electronic data interchange, such as the credit card industry, many parties viewed EDI as having little impact on fraud beyond transplanting the problem from paper to the computer — a perception that has proved wrong.

Moreover, notwithstanding the administrative cost-saving features of EDI, the conversion to a paperless claim environment poses significant risks. Unless the risks are addressed in payers' electronic claims systems, they will significantly enhance the ability of unscrupulous individuals to commit fraud through creation of fraudulent accounts or the ability to test payer limits or guidelines on a real-time basis.

Accordingly, payers who implement EDI without due consideration of EDI's anti-fraud implications will fail to capitalize on any enhanced long-term ability to fight fraud. In fact, they may find themselves far more vulnerable to fraud in the electronic world than they were in the paper environment.

On the flip side, technology in fact may be the key to fraud detection in the future. Most importantly, technology allows payers to find the most likely perpetrators of health care fraud and detect fraud before money is paid out.

EDI systems should help, for example, by virtue of the standardized electronic claim forms and the data sets that insurers will be able to derive from their universe of claims data. Using sophisticated technology, payers can compare provider practices using the provider's own claims data, which allows the payers to evaluate whether specific professional behavior warrants additional review.

The task for those that pay for health care is to take the extensive experience in fighting fraud in a paper environment and convert those indicators to EDI.

To the extent possible, EDI systems must be designed to compensate — through built-in system edits — for the loss of the collective experience and instinct of human claims personnel. Such edits may be as simple as isolating claims for non-emergency services rendered on Sundays or holidays, or as complicated as system protocols that identify inconsistencies between treatments billed and patient diagnoses.

Understanding how paper-claim fraud indicators work today and developing comparable system edits in the EDI environment will be the critical task for system designers in the years to come.

EDI systems also expose payers to several new and increased risks. For example, the very efficiency and speed of EDI transactions will make payers more vulnerable to entrepreneurial fraud schemes in which perpetrators find themselves able to tap a payer's electronic system for an immediate "big score," and then drop from sight long before any retrospective detection method brings the crime to light.

Similarly, because EDI systems require payers to link their computer systems to those of a wide variety of external parties — including individual providers, electronic claims clearinghouses and financial institutions — there will be increased opportunities for fraud by parties to the transactions, making payers' systems more vulnerable to external attack by criminal computer "hackers."

The electronic medium also can make fraud look easier to commit and get away with because EDI eliminates paper evidentiary documents and creates a relative ease and perceived anonymity of "touch-of-a-button" computer crimes.

Tackling the Task Ahead

Private payers continue to be a leading force in the fight against health care fraud. With the dramatic changes ahead in the health care marketplace and regulatory environment, the challenges in this area have only just begun.

Medicare Beneficiary Advisory Bulletin on HMOs

This Advisory Bulletin is issued by the U.S. Department of Health and Human Services' Office of Inspector General and the Health Care Financing Administration's Office of Managed Care. It addresses issues related to HMO enrollment, the provision of services, and the disenrollment of Medicare program beneficiaries.

The Office of Inspector General was established by Congress to find and eliminate fraud, waste and abuse. It issues Special Fraud Alerts and Advisory Bulletins to show Medicare beneficiaries where and how to look for potential problems. The Health Care Financing Administration's Office of Managed Care works to ensure that Medicare beneficiaries are given quality health care in their HMO plans.

Know Your Rights

INTRODUCTION

If you are thinking of joining a Medicare contracting health maintenance organization (HMO), or are enrolled in an HMO, this advisory bulletin gives you important information. In addition, this bulletin also tells you how you can get help and where you can make complaints if you believe any of your rights have been violated or the HMO has acted inappropriately.

What Are Medicare Contracting HMOs?

Medicare contracts with HMOs to provide a full range of Medicare benefits to you. **Medicare contracting HMOs must give you all the health care services that are covered under the Medicare program, except hospice services** (See your Medicare Handbook for specific details). In addition, HMOs may offer additional benefits, either at no charge or for an additional charge.

There are two types of Medicare contracting HMOs - **risk HMOs** and **cost HMOs.** Most HMOs are risk HMOs, and **this bulletin deals exclusively with risk HMOs**[1].

[1]You should find out whether the HMO you are considering joining is a risk or cost HMO. If it is a cost HMO, be sure to request additional information about the operation and benefits associated with this type of plan. Some of the issues raised in this bulletin may also apply to cost HMOs.

In general, if you enroll in a **risk HMO plan**, sometimes called a health plan or plan:

- You must get all of your medical care through the plan's doctors, hospitals, skilled nursing facilities, home health agencies, and other health care providers. You are "locked-in" to receive care through your HMO plan. You may, however, get emergency care and unforseen out-of-area urgently needed care, when necessary, from non-plan providers. Some plans may offer a **point-of-service option** which allows members to use non-plan providers in certain cases.
- You must select a primary care doctor participating in the plan. This doctor is responsible for coordinating your care. You must obtain a referral from this doctor in order to see a specialist or obtain other services through the plan.

Part I: Enrollment and Disenrollment Rights

ENROLLMENT RIGHTS

When you are considering enrolling in an HMO, the HMO:

- Must provide you with complete and accurate information;
- Must enroll you without regard to your health status;
- Must not offer you gifts or other financial inducements to encourage you to enroll.

Complete and Accurate Information

Before you decide to enroll in a plan, HMO sales, marketing or other plan representatives must give you complete and accurate information about the benefits and the services their HMO provides.

Make sure the HMO representative tells you whether the HMO offers any additional benefits besides those benefits covered under the Medicare program. If so, there may be limits on how often you can use the benefits or how much the HMO will pay for them.

For example, if you take prescription drugs, you should ask the plan before you enroll if the drugs you take are covered. If the drugs are covered, ask about whether there are limits to the coverage and whether you are required to use certain pharmacies. [**NOTE:** Many plans do not cover all prescription drugs. Plans may set a maximum dollar amount on the drugs they cover each quarter or each year.]

In addition, the HMO representative must tell you if the HMO requires copayments for any services, including drugs, and the amount of such copayments. [**NOTE:** Additional benefits and copayments may change each year.]

Make sure that sales, marketing or other plan representatives tell you about how their HMO operates and about all HMO providers and facilities that will be available to you in your area. This includes the home health agencies and skilled nursing facilities associated with their HMO. Make sure you understand if there are any limitations on using the HMO-affiliated providers. For example, certain hospitals may only be used for special services such as transplants. Some doctors may only work at certain hospitals or with certain specialists.

Make sure you understand which primary care doctors will accept you as a new patient. Some doctors may not be accepting new patients. Also make sure you understand under what circumstances and how frequently you can change primary care doctors and what happens if any of your doctors leave the plan. In addition, sales, marketing and other plan representatives must tell you that you will be **"locked-in"** to the HMO and its providers once you enroll and what this will mean to you.

Sales, marketing and other plan representatives must tell you that when you enroll in a risk HMO, you cannot continue to use any of your current doctors or hospitals unless they are affiliated directly with the HMO.

If your current doctor is affiliated with the HMO, you still need to be sure that he or she can accept you as an HMO patient.

If you should choose to go to a doctor or hospital not affiliated with your plan, you will have to pay the entire bill yourself.

Sales, marketing and other plan representatives must clearly and accurately describe, and must not misrepresent, HMO benefits and services.

Medicare law prohibits HMO representatives from enrolling you in an HMO without your permission.

- **You are not required to sign any HMO forms unless you are enrolling in an HMO. If a sales representative gives you a form to sign and you are not sure what it is, do not sign it.**
- **Do not give the HMO your Medicare or Social Security number unless you are enrolling.**
- **HMO marketing representatives are not allowed to come to your home unless you have given them permission in advance. This restriction applies to any personal residence, including your room in a nursing home, rest home or assisted living arrangement.**

If you received false, misleading or incomplete information, then you may have been improperly enrolled in an HMO. If so, you have the right to be retroactively disenrolled and to return to traditional Medicare coverage, or to enroll in another HMO. [**NOTE**: Of course, you can disenroll from an HMO at any time. See Disenrollment Rights section. Also, enrolling in a new Medicare HMO automatically disenrolls you from your current HMO.]

Enrollment Without Health Screenings

An HMO must enroll all eligible Medicare beneficiaries who want to enroll, regardless of their age, health status or the amount or cost of the health services needed.

HMOs are not allowed to make you undergo a health screening before you enroll. **Pre-enrollment health screening or questions about your health or physical status are against the law.** These screenings can be used by the HMO to identify sick beneficiaries and those with chronic conditions, and to discourage them from enrolling. [**NOTE**: There are two exceptions to the rule about health screening before enrollment. An HMO can ask you whether you are receiving kidney dialysis or have received a kidney transplant, or whether you are receiving hospice services. If you are receiving these services or have these conditions, you can not enroll in an HMO.]

Before you enroll, sales, marketing or other HMO plan representatives should not ask:

- **how often you visit the doctor;**
- **how many doctors you have;**
- **how many times you have been hospitalized in the last year;**
- **whether you have any conditions for which you take medicine on a regular basis, or;**
- **whether you exercise regularly.**

Also be alert for improper screenings when an HMO requires or offers:

- **free physical exams before enrollment;**
- **free screening or diagnostic tests at health fairs or at marketing presentations.**

In addition, watch for sales, marketing or other HMO plan representatives who tell you that the HMO would not be a good choice for you because (1) referrals to specialists would be limited, (2) you might have to wait for services, or (3) services would be more limited in an HMO.

After you enroll, the HMO may ask you questions, give you questionnaires to fill out, or give you a physical exam to assist them in providing your care.

Enrollment Without Being Offered Free Gifts or Other Inducements

It is illegal for an HMO to offer you free gifts or incentives to get you or anyone else to enroll in an HMO.

HMOs are not allowed to offer you free gifts to encourage you to enroll or as a reward for attending marketing presentations. They are not allowed to offer incentives to get you to recommend them to your friends either. These incentives are not allowed because they could affect your decision to enroll or to recommend that a friend enroll. It's okay for the HMO to offer promotional materials worth less than $10, such as key chains, mugs and calendars, as well as light refreshments at a marketing presentation, as long as these are given to everyone regardless of their decision to enroll.

DISENROLLMENT RIGHTS

Disenrollment Is Your Decision

Once you are enrolled in an HMO, you may wish to disenroll at some point. Whether you stay enrolled in or leave an HMO, it is your decision. Your HMO cannot try to keep you from disenrolling nor can the HMO try to get you to leave.

When You Decide to Leave Your HMO

HMOs must process written requests for disenrollment in a timely manner.

HMOs may not delay, withhold disenrollment information or forms, or otherwise make it hard for you to disenroll from a plan. If you want to disenroll from your HMO because you are unhappy or dissatisfied with services, or for any other reason, your

HMO should help you disenroll. You must submit a written request to disenroll, and the HMO should help you complete any necessary paperwork. [**NOTE**: Whoever has authority under State law to make health care decisions for you can enroll you in or disenroll you from an HMO.] You may also go to a Social Security office to disenroll from your HMO.

Make sure your HMO tells you the date when your disenrollment is effective. It is usually the first day of the month following receipt of your disenrollment request. If you get services from a non-HMO provider when you are still a member of your HMO, neither your HMO nor Medicare will pay.

[**NOTE**: If you disenroll from a HMO and have any pre-existing medical conditions, many Medicare supplemental insurance (Medigap) policies will not sell you a policy or will impose a waiting period for those conditions. That means you could be without supplemental insurance coverage for that condition for a period of time unless you enroll in another HMO. Also, some Medigap policies only have open enrollment periods once a year. Remember to look for a policy that will provide coverage for your pre-existing conditions, and will be available when you disenroll.]

If Your HMO Encourages You to Disenroll

The premiums that your HMO gets from the Medicare program are designed to reimburse the plan for all the covered services you need. **The HMO is not allowed to try to get you to leave or to delay or deny you**

services because you need heart surgery, transplants, long term nursing or rehabilitative services or other expensive treatments.

Your HMO must not encourage you to disenroll:

- **Because it will be expensive to treat your condition or meet your medical needs.**
- **By delaying expensive medical care for a long time, or by denying such care.**
- **By telling you that you can re-enroll in the HMO after you have received the necessary high cost services outside the HMO.**

Unless you enroll in another HMO, if you disenroll from the HMO to get a specific service or procedure, you will have to pay any deductibles or coinsurance under the payment rules of the traditional Medicare program.

Part II: Your Rights to Medical Services in an HMO

This part addresses your rights to medical services and benefits in a Medicare contracting HMO once you are enrolled.

Your Rights To Services

When you are enrolled in an HMO, you have a right to:

- **Medically necessary care in a timely manner.**
- **Emergency medical care and unforseen out-of-area urgent care.**

Your HMO must provide all medically necessary covered services. Covered services include all the benefits provided under the Medicare program and any additional services offered by the HMO.

Your HMO must have enough qualified primary care and specialty care doctors, as well as other health care providers and facilities, to provide you with all medically necessary covered services. If the HMO does not have enough qualified providers, it must arrange for services to be provided to you outside the plan at no extra cost to you.

HMOs must make necessary medical care and services available and accessible to you. The HMO may not:

- **Create or permit delays like repeated busy signals when you call to make appointments;**
- **Make you wait an unreasonably long time for appointments;**
- **Unreasonably restrict the days or hours that you may be seen by the plan's providers;**
- **Create or permit unreasonable delays in arranging for surgery, hospitalization or other services by using review or approval mechanisms;**
- **Inappropriately deny or limit referrals to specialists in or outside the plan;**
- **Unreasonably limit the amount of nursing home, home health or therapy services.**

Getting Emergency and Out-of-Area Care

Your HMO must pay for emergency care and for unforseen, urgently needed, out-of-area care you get from non-HMO health care providers, including necessary follow-up care.

Emergency Care

Emergencies are situations when you need medical care immediately because of sudden or suddenly worsening illness or injury, and the time needed to reach your plan doctor or hospital appears to you to risk permanent damage to your health.

Your HMO must not:

- **Tell you that you can only get emergency care through its doctors and at its facilities;**
- **Require you to get prior authorization for emergency services;**
- **Deny your claim for emergency services after you get the services, because what appeared to be an emergency condition turned out not to be an emergency condition.**

If you believe you have an emergency, you may seek emergency care outside the plan and the HMO must cover and pay for those emergency services you got from the outside provider. Your HMO must pay for all procedures performed during the evaluation and treatment of your emergency condition, unless those services were completely unrelated to the emergency condition. If possible, you should call (or have someone call) your HMO as soon as possible when receiving emergency care.

[**NOTE**: You should be aware that hospitals are required by law to provide screening for emergency medical conditions. If necessary, hospitals must provide stabilizing treatment or arrange for an appropriate transfer to another facility, whether or not your HMO authorizes these services. The hospital may not refuse to provide emergency services to you because your HMO will not authorize such services.]

Out-of-Area Urgent Care

Urgent care situations are when you have an unexpected illness or injury while you are temporarily outside the HMO's service area. Your HMO must pay for your urgent care if:

- **Your illness or injury is unexpected; and**
- **You are temporarily away from the HMO service area; and**
- **Your illness or injury requires medical care which cannot be delayed until you return home.**

If possible, you should call (or have someone call) your HMO as soon as possible when receiving out-of-area urgent care.

Transfers From Another Facility

If you have received emergency or urgent care services from a non-HMO facility, your HMO may not attempt to transfer you back to its own facility from another facility outside its plan before the non-HMO facility decides that your condition is stabilized.

Coverage of Follow-Up Care

Your HMO must cover all medically necessary follow-up care related to your emergency condition, or unforseen out-of-area urgent care, provided outside the plan if that care cannot be delayed without adverse medical effects to you.

Part III:
How to Make a Complaint

You should be aware that you and your HMO may disagree about what care is medically necessary.

You have the right to appeal if you believe that medically necessary care has been denied, reduced or terminated inappropriately.

Here are some examples of situations in which you have the right to appeal:

- **Your doctor does not prescribe covered treatments or tests, refer you to a specialist, or does not admit you for hospital services you believe you need;**
- **Your HMO refuses to authorize or provide tests, treatments or referrals recommended by your primary care doctor;**
- **Your HMO does not authorize a second opinion on the need for surgery. (Second opinions are a Medicare covered benefit.)**
- **Your HMO or your doctor decides to reduce or terminate services you are already receiving, such as home health care or physical therapy, or decides to discharge you from a nursing home;**
- **You encounter an unreasonable delay or difficulty in arranging for surgery, hospitalization, tests, doctor visits or any other needed services, and you believe this is a way of denying you care;**

- **Your HMO will not pay your claims for emergency care or out-of-area urgent care you received from a non-HMO provider;**
- **A decision is made to discharge you from a hospital before you believe you are ready to be discharged.** [NOTE: When you are in the hospital and your HMO decides that you do not need to be there any longer, you can ask for immediate review by a Peer Review Organization (PRO). If you ask for an immediate review, you can stay in the hospital at no charge during the review. The review usually takes at least 24 hours.]

The Appeals Process

Your HMO is required to notify you when it **denies, reduces, or terminates services or payment for services.** (Whether or not you have written notification, you may appeal.) The HMO must also provide you with written information about your appeal rights and the process you must follow, including time frames for each step.

The appeals process begins with your written request to the HMO asking it to review the denial, reduction or termination. If the HMO does not reverse its decision, the appeal automatically goes next to an independent review organization that contracts with Medicare to review HMO denials. If the review organization does not decide fully in your favor, you may request a hearing from Medicare.

If you need help in deciding whether to appeal, or if you have questions regarding what you must do to appeal, you can contact your local or State Insurance Counselling and Assistance (ICA) Program. Call the Medicare Hot Line at 1-800-638-6833 to get the number of the ICA in your area.

Complaints About Quality

If you have complaints about the quality of care you have received by your HMO or any of its providers, including hospitals, skilled nursing facilities and home health agencies, you can complain to your HMO or a Peer Review Organization (PRO). PROs are groups of doctors and health care professionals that monitor the quality of care provided to Medicare beneficiaries. Call the Medicare Hot Line or your ICA to get the number of the PRO serving your area (See ***Part IV: Where to Go For Help***). The PRO will investigate your complaint.

Other Complaints

If you have other complaints about the HMO, such as physician demeanor or adequacy of the facilities, contact your HMO directly. Your HMO must have written procedures, including time frames, for investigating these types of complaints (also called grievances). The HMO representatives will review these complaints and notify you in writing of their conclusions.

Part IV: Where to Go for Help

What you need to do if you believe your HMO is not meeting its obligations or may be violating your rights:

- Complain directly to the HMO. You must write to your HMO asking it to reconsider its decision to deny, reduce or terminate care, coverage or payment. Every HMO is required to have a process to handle complaints, and the HMO must give you detailed information on how to file a complaint.
- Contact your local or State Insurance Counselling and Assistance Program (ICA) which has been set up to assist Medicare beneficiaries in resolving problems with, or answering questions about, their Medicare benefits. To obtain the phone number of your ICA, you can call the Medicare toll-free Hot Line at **1-800-638-6833** or your local area Agency on Aging office. To obtain the number of your local aging office, you can call **1-800-677-1116** (the Eldercare locator number).
- Contact the HHS Office of Inspector General through its toll-free Hot Line at **1-800-HHS-TIPS** (1-800-447-8477), or contact the HCFA Medicare toll-free Hot Line at **1-800-638-6833**. Contacting one of these offices about improper practices will not resolve your individual problem, but may help to stop any improper practices.

QUIZ YOURSELF

There are several important questions you should ask yourself regarding HMO participation.

Do you know:

- What lock-in means?
- The role of your primary care doctor?
- How the HMO's referral process works?
- The HMO's rules and responsibilities about paying for emergency and out-of-area urgent care?
- Whether HMO enrollment is a good choice for you if you travel or are out of the HMO service area for long periods of time?
- How to disenroll from an HMO?
- How to complain if you have a problem?